Leon Prado

Oníric Control
A Dream Traveler's Manual

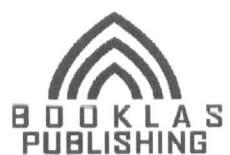

Original Title: *Oníric Control: A Dream Traveler's Manual*
Copyright © 2024, published by Luiz Antonio dos Santos ME.
This book is a non-fiction work that explores the practice and concepts of lucid dreaming. Through a comprehensive approach, the author provides practical tools for achieving awareness and control within dreams, unlocking the potential for self-discovery, creativity, and personal transformation.
2st Edition
Production Team
Author: Leon Prado
Editor: Luiz Santos
Cover: Studios Booklas / Ethan Graves
Consultant: Miranda Keats
Researchers: Thomas Varela, Sophia Mendez, Rafael Quinn
Layout Designer: Oliver Strauss,
Publication and Identification
Oníric Control: A Dream Traveler's Manual
Booklas, 2024
Categories: Psychology / Consciousness Studies / Personal Development
DDC: 154.632 – **CDU:** 159.93
All rights reserved to:
Luiz Antonio dos Santos ME / Booklas
No part of this book may be reproduced, stored in a retrieval system, or transmitted by any means—electronic, mechanical, photocopying, recording, or otherwise—without prior written permission from the copyright holder.

Summary

Systematic Index 5
Prologue 10
Chapter 1 The World of Dreams 13
Chapter 2 The Nature of Dream Consciousness 20
Chapter 3 The Benefits of Controlling Your Dreams 25
Chapter 4 Myths and Realities About Lucid Dreaming 30
Chapter 5 Sleep and Dream Cycles 35
Chapter 6 How the Brain Creates Dreams 40
Chapter 7 The Science of Lucid Dreaming 45
Chapter 8 Dreams in History and Mythology 50
Chapter 9 Dream Incubation in Ancient Cultures 55
Chapter 10 Dreams in Eastern Spiritual Traditions 60
Chapter 11 Shamanic and Indigenous Perspectives on Dreams . 65
Chapter 12 Lucid Dreaming in the Modern Era 72
Chapter 13 Preparing for the Oneiric Journey 78
Chapter 14 Keeping a Dream Journal 83
Chapter 15 Improving Dream Recall 88
Chapter 16 Dream Signs and Personal Patterns 93
Chapter 17 Reality Checks 98
Chapter 18 Dream Incubation and Intention 103
Chapter 19 Mnemonic Induction of Lucid Dreaming 108
Chapter 20 The WBTB Technique 113
Chapter 21 Wake-Initiated Lucid Dreaming (WILD) 118
Chapter 22 Other Induction Techniques and Tools 123

Chapter 23 The First Lucid Dreaming Experience 129
Chapter 24 Staying Lucid 134
Chapter 25 Navigation and Control in the Oneiric Environment
.... 139
Chapter 26 Transforming Fears 144
Chapter 27 Healing and Personal Growth................................. 149
Chapter 28 Creativity and Problem-Solving............................. 154
Chapter 29 Spiritual Exploration in Dreams............................. 158
Chapter 30 Tibetan Dream Yoga in Practice 163
Chapter 31 Out-of-Body Experiences.. 168
Chapter 32 Integrating Dream and Reality 173
Chapter 33 Dream Mastery and Next Steps.............................. 178
Epilogue 183

Systematic Index

Chapter 1: The World of Dreams - Explores humanity's historical and cultural relationship with dreams, discussing various interpretations and the potential for lucid dreaming.

Chapter 2: The Nature of Dream Consciousness - Discusses the differences between waking and dream consciousness, the phenomenon of lucid dreaming, and the potential for training dream lucidity.

Chapter 3: The Benefits of Controlling Your Dreams - Details the advantages of lucid dreaming, including overcoming nightmares, enhancing creativity, promoting self-awareness, and improving mental health.

Chapter 4: Myths and Realities About Lucid Dreaming - Clarifies common misconceptions about lucid dreaming, addressing fears and doubts while emphasizing its natural and safe nature.

Chapter 5: Sleep and Dream Cycles - Explains the different stages of sleep, including non-REM and REM sleep, and how understanding these cycles can enhance lucid dreaming practices.

Chapter 6: How the Brain Creates Dreams - Details the brain activity during REM sleep and how it contributes to the creation of dreams, including the roles of the amygdala, hippocampus, and prefrontal cortex.

Chapter 7: The Science of Lucid Dreaming - Explores the scientific evidence behind lucid dreaming, discussing key experiments, brain activity during lucid dreams, and potential applications.

Chapter 8: Dreams in History and Mythology - Examines the historical and mythological significance of dreams across various cultures, from ancient civilizations to Eastern spiritual traditions.

Chapter 9: Dream Incubation in Ancient Cultures - Discusses the ancient practice of dream incubation, where individuals sought specific dream experiences for guidance, healing, or problem-solving.

Chapter 10: Dreams in Eastern Spiritual Traditions - Explores how Eastern spiritual traditions like Buddhism, Hinduism, Taoism, and Zen Buddhism view and utilize dreams for spiritual growth and understanding.

Chapter 11: Shamanic and Indigenous Perspectives on Dreams - Details how indigenous cultures and shamanic traditions view dreams as connections to the spiritual world, used for guidance, healing, and community well-being.

Chapter 12: Lucid Dreaming in the Modern Era - Traces the evolution of lucid dreaming from esoteric interest to a scientifically studied and applied practice for personal development.

Chapter 13: Preparing for the Oneiric Journey - Provides guidance on how to prepare for lucid dreaming through environmental adjustments, healthy habits, and mental conditioning.

Chapter 14: Keeping a Dream Journal - Emphasizes the importance of recording dreams to enhance recall, recognize patterns, and facilitate lucid dreaming.

Chapter 15: Improving Dream Recall - Offers techniques and strategies to improve the ability to remember dreams, which is crucial for lucid dreaming practice.

Chapter 16: Dream Signs and Personal Patterns - Explains how to identify recurring symbols and patterns in dreams, which can serve as triggers for recognizing the dream state.

Chapter 17: Reality Checks - Details the use of reality checks to test whether one is dreaming, training the mind to question its state of consciousness.

Chapter 18: Dream Incubation and Intention - Explores the technique of dream incubation, using intention and pre-sleep suggestions to influence dream content and achieve specific goals within dreams.

Chapter 19: Mnemonic Induction of Lucid Dreaming - Details the MILD technique, which uses prospective memory and intention to increase the likelihood of lucid dreams.

Chapter 20: The WBTB Technique - Describes the Wake Back to Bed (WBTB) technique, which involves interrupting sleep and then returning to it to increase the chances of lucid dreaming.

Chapter 21: Wake-Initiated Lucid Dreaming (WILD) - Explores the WILD technique, which aims to enter a lucid dream directly from the waking state by maintaining awareness while the body falls asleep.

Chapter 22: Other Induction Techniques and Tools - Discusses various alternative techniques and tools for inducing lucid dreams, including sensory triggers, meditation practices, and supplements.

Chapter 23: The First Lucid Dreaming Experience - Describes the typical first experiences of lucid dreaming, including emotional responses and strategies for stabilizing lucidity.

Chapter 24: Staying Lucid - Provides techniques for maintaining lucidity within a dream, including sensory engagement, movement, and mental commands.

Chapter 25: Navigation and Control in the Oneiric Environment - Discusses how to navigate and control the dream environment, including movement, manipulation of objects, and interaction with dream characters.

Chapter 26: Transforming Fears - Explores how lucid dreaming can be used to confront and transform fears and nightmares, changing the dreamer's relationship with fear.

Chapter 27: Healing and Personal Growth - Details how lucid dreaming can be used for emotional healing, self-discovery, and personal development by exploring and reframing unconscious content.

Chapter 28: Creativity and Problem-Solving - Discusses the use of lucid dreaming to enhance creativity, solve problems, and improve skills by accessing the mind's boundless potential.

Chapter 29: Spiritual Exploration in Dreams - Explores the use of lucid dreams for spiritual exploration, including encounters with guides, experiences of unity, and seeking answers to existential questions.

Chapter 30: Tibetan Dream Yoga in Practice - Details Dream Yoga as a path to self-discovery and spiritual development, emphasizing lucidity as a means to awaken to the true nature of mind and reality.

Chapter 31: Out-of-Body Experiences - Explores out-of-body experiences (OBEs) and their challenge to the boundaries between subjective perception and objective reality.

Chapter 32: Integrating Dream and Reality - Discusses integrating lucidity from dreams into daily life, transforming everyday perception, and recognizing the fluid relationship between dream and reality.

Chapter 33: Dream Mastery and Next Steps - Concludes the exploration of lucid dreaming as a continuous journey of self-discovery, emphasizing the importance of practice, mindfulness, and using dreams for personal growth.

Prologue

The sensation of controlling one's dreams is beyond words. Only those who have experienced it, who have dared to open their eyes within their own minds, truly understand the magnitude of this power. We are all chained to a single reality – or so we have been led to believe. But what if there were another path? A hidden portal between sleep and wakefulness, a secret door leading to a universe where anything is possible?

The human mind, that unfathomable enigma, operates under rules that few comprehend. In our waking state, we are prisoners of logic, hostages to gravity, subjected to the immutable laws of matter. But when our eyes close, and we plunge into dreams, the chains are broken. There, time is malleable. Space bends. Identity dissolves. Yet, most people traverse this passage like castaways adrift, unaware of their own ability to take the helm and steer their vessel.

The central question isn't whether it's possible to awaken within a dream, but why we haven't been taught this. Ancient traditions knew this secret. Shamans, Tibetan monks, Egyptian priests, and mystics of all eras understood that dreams are more than random projections of the mind – they are maps to other dimensions of consciousness. For millennia, techniques have been developed to pierce the veil of the unconscious and achieve lucidity within one's own dreams. This knowledge was passed down as a closely guarded secret, but it has reached us. And it is before you now.

Most dreamers are controlled *by* their dreams. They plunge into bizarre scenarios, relive distorted memories, face nightmares, and wake up sweating, never realizing they could have transformed each of those moments. The overwhelming nightmare that makes the heart race can be transmuted into ecstasy. The monster that pursues can kneel like a master in reverence. The abyss that opens beneath one's feet can be converted into the ultimate experience of freedom – flight. The key to this transmutation lies in mastering the oníric mind.

Have you ever felt that sudden clarity within a dream? A flash of awareness where you realized, even for a fleeting moment, that nothing there was real? That fleeting moment, in which you almost managed to direct events, but soon lost yourself in the fog of the unconscious? This sensation need not be an accident. It can be cultivated, trained, and refined until it becomes a natural state.

And when that happens, what was once just a confused landscape becomes a vast territory to be explored. Every door can lead to a new universe. Every thought can shape the landscape. You can fly over endless mountains, create entire cities with the power of imagination, converse with wise ancestors, or transcend the limits of the possible. Within the lucid dream, there are no barriers. There is only will – and what it can manifest.

But the true power of oníric control goes beyond the euphoria of flying or creating worlds. It touches something deeper. The subconscious mind, that great architect of reality, operates silently, influencing every thought, every choice, every emotion. Dreams are its language. By understanding it, you not only unlock the oníric universe – you rewrite your own waking reality. Like a stone thrown into a lake, the changes made in the dream world reverberate, shaping your mind, your perceptions, and ultimately, your very life.

Modern science is beginning to confirm what the ancients already knew: by learning to become lucid in dreams, you expand your self-awareness, strengthen creativity, improve your problem-solving abilities, and access deeper layers of the psyche. What you learn within the dream doesn't just stay in the dream. It translates into mental clarity, emotional balance, and a new perspective on the waking world.

Are you ready to cross this threshold?

This work is not just a manual. It is an invitation to the most extraordinary journey a human being can undertake: the conscious exploration of one's own mind. The path has been traced. The keys are here. The ancient knowledge, now backed by science, awaits the one who desires to awaken.

The question now is not whether dreams can be controlled, the question is: are you ready to take that control?

Luiz Santos Editor

Chapter 1
The World of Dreams

Humanity's relationship with dreams spans the centuries, blending mystery, fascination, and a relentless pursuit of understanding. In every age and culture, dreams have been interpreted in various ways: as divine messages, manifestations of the unconscious, or even portals to other realities. Today, science has made significant advances in attempting to decipher this phenomenon, but even with all the accumulated technology and knowledge, dreams continue to hold unfathomable secrets. More than mere random projections of the sleeping mind, they represent a state of consciousness that defies waking logic, creating scenarios, emotions, and experiences that often seem as real as waking reality itself.

Among these mysteries, one of the most intriguing is the possibility of becoming conscious within one's own dream. This experience, called lucid dreaming, is not limited to a sporadic or random phenomenon, but rather a skill that can be cultivated and improved. When a dreamer realizes that they are inside a dream, they acquire a level of control that allows them to explore this inner universe with freedom and intention. This means not only recognizing the dream as an alternate state of mind, but also actively interacting with it, transforming scenarios, experiencing sensations impossible in the waking world, and even seeking answers to profound personal questions. What was once considered a rare phenomenon or restricted to a few individuals is now widely studied and accessible to anyone willing to train their mind to achieve this form of consciousness.

The exploration of lucid dreams opens doors to a vast field of possibilities, from self-knowledge to creativity and spiritual growth. Some ancient cultures already recognized this practice as a powerful tool, while modern science is beginning to unravel the brain mechanisms that make this experience possible. Understanding dreams is not just an intellectual exercise, but a journey towards mastery of one's own mind. The ability to awaken within the dream, to perceive that everything there is the fruit of one's own imagination and, yet, to be able to fully experience it, challenges the boundaries between the real and the illusory. The study and practice of lucid dreams not only provide fascinating experiences, but also help to expand the limits of human consciousness, allowing the dreamer to become the architect of their own oníric universe.

Imagine, for a moment, being inside a dream and knowing you are dreaming. Knowing that nothing around you is real in the physical sense, but that you can interact, transform scenarios, and even fly if you wish. This experience, known as a lucid dream, is not only possible – it is a trainable skill.

In this book, we will explore in depth how to develop this ability, but first, it is essential to understand why we dream and how different cultures have viewed dreams throughout history. The purpose of this chapter is to open the doors to this journey, showing that mastering one's own dreams can be more than just a pastime: it can be a powerful tool for self-knowledge, creativity, and even spiritual growth.

What Are Dreams?

Dreaming is a universal experience. Every night, our minds create vivid stories, often absurd, and transport us to realities where the laws of physics and logic become malleable. But what exactly is a dream?

From a neuroscientific perspective, dreams are products of brain activity during sleep, especially in the REM (Rapid Eye Movement) phase. In this state, areas of the brain associated with emotion and memory become highly active, while the part responsible for logical thinking – the prefrontal cortex – reduces its activity. This explains why we accept illogical situations as normal within dreams.

On the other hand, in various cultures, dreams have been seen as divine messages, spiritual journeys, or portals to other planes of existence. For the ancient Egyptians, they were messages from the gods. For the Greeks, a means of predicting the future. For shamans, a bridge between the physical and spiritual worlds.

Regardless of the approach, the fact is that dreams have a significant impact on the human psyche. They reflect fears, desires, and unconscious aspects of the mind. And when we manage to realize that we are dreaming – acquiring oníric lucidity – we begin to consciously interact with this universe, instead of just being carried away by it.

The idea of controlling one's own dreams may seem too fantastic to some, but studies indicate that approximately 50% of people have had at least one spontaneous lucid dream. This means that this experience is not something rare or unattainable, but rather a natural extension of human consciousness.

If the brain already has this ability to realize that it is dreaming occasionally, what prevents someone from learning to do it deliberately? The answer lies in training. Just like learning a new language or playing an instrument, oníric lucidity can be developed with practice and appropriate techniques.

Before delving into these techniques – which will be covered in the following chapters – it is essential to prepare the mind. The first shift in perspective is to realize that dreams are not just fleeting illusions, but rather a legitimate state of consciousness. Just as we live our waking hours with attention and intention, we can also "wake up" within dreams and take the reins of the experience.

This change in mindset is essential, as many people treat dreams as something irrelevant, forgetting them upon waking. But those who develop the ability to remember, analyze, and interact with their dreams discover a new world of possibilities.

The quest for understanding dreams is not recent. Since time immemorial, different civilizations have recognized their importance. The Sumerians, the first great civilization in history, recorded dreams on clay tablets more than 4,000 years ago. The ancient Egyptians had priests specialized in interpreting dreams, believing that they brought messages from the gods.

In Ancient Greece, healing temples known as dream incubatories were places where people slept in the hope of receiving divine revelations. Aristotle was one of the first to suggest that dreams could be generated by the mind, and not just sent by higher entities.

In the Tibetan Buddhist tradition, the practice of Dream Yoga teaches that recognizing the illusion of dreams can help to perceive the illusion of reality, promoting a higher state of consciousness.

Throughout the centuries, this duality between the mystical and scientific view of dreams has persisted. But with the advancement of neuroscience, many of the ancient beliefs have begun to find support in science. Today, we know that dreams have essential functions for the mind, such as consolidating memories, processing emotions, and even simulating future scenarios.

The ability to become conscious within a dream is not just a scientific curiosity or a mental trick – it can bring real benefits.

Overcoming Nightmares: Nightmares can be distressing experiences, but in a lucid dream, the dreamer can face them without fear, knowing that nothing there can hurt them. This can help in overcoming trauma and anxiety.

Stimulating Creativity: Many artists, writers, and inventors report having had innovative ideas in dreams. Salvador Dalí, for example, used techniques to capture oníric images and incorporate them into his art. In lucid dreams, this creative exploration becomes even more powerful.

Self-Knowledge: Dreams reflect deep contents of the mind. By consciously interacting with them, we can explore aspects of our inner self, understand repressed emotions, and gain insights into our lives.

Unlimited Experiences: Within a lucid dream, the laws of physics do not apply. We can fly, walk through walls, visit exotic places, and create entire worlds at will. It is an experience of absolute freedom.

Improved Sleep Quality. Contrary to What People may think, lucid dreams training does not harm the rest. It may improve it. Studies show that lucid dreamers will develop a more positive relationship with sleep, reducing nightmare incidents and promoting a more restorative rest.

This book will not only teach how to induce lucid dreams, but also show how to use them in the best possible way. We will explore everything from the fundamentals of sleep and consciousness to practical techniques for achieving lucidity, stabilizing it, and making the most of each oníric experience.

In the following chapters, we will delve deeper into the nature of oníric consciousness, understand the difference between ordinary dreams and lucid dreams, and see how science proves this phenomenon.

The journey that begins here is not just about controlling dreams – it is about expanding consciousness and discovering that there is much more to the universe of the mind than we imagine.

If you have ever dreamed that you were flying, exploring unknown lands, or talking to mysterious figures, you may have felt a glimpse of the unlimited potential that dreams offer. Now, imagine being able to do this consciously, whenever you wish.

Chapter 2
The Nature of Dream Consciousness

To understand what it means to be conscious within a dream, we first need to understand what consciousness itself *is*. During our waking hours, we're accustomed to perceiving the world in a continuous flow, analyzing information, making decisions, and reflecting on our own existence. However, when we sleep, this clarity vanishes, and the mind surrenders to dream narratives that we accept without question, no matter how absurd they may be.

Dream consciousness is different from waking consciousness. In an ordinary dream, we go with the flow of events without realizing we're dreaming. The scenery can change suddenly, characters can appear out of nowhere, time can warp – and yet, our minds accept it all as normal. This happens because, in the sleep state, the brain operates differently. The prefrontal cortex, responsible for critical thinking and logical reasoning, reduces its activity, while areas associated with emotion and memory become more active. This makes the dream seem real and immersive, but it also explains why we rarely question its veracity while we're inside it.

When we talk about lucid dreams, we're talking about a phenomenon that occurs when the critical part of the brain reactivates within the dream itself. Suddenly, the dreamer perceives the illusion and regains the ability to question what they see around them. This inner awakening doesn't necessarily mean total control of the dream experience, but it's the first step. It's possible to be lucid within a dream and still not be able to shape it easily. In many cases, the person realizes they're dreaming but continues to be carried along by the dream's plot, without actively intervening.

The experience of lucidity varies from person to person. Some report a sudden moment of clarity, as if a veil has been lifted, while others enter a state of gradual lucidity, where the unreality of the dream becomes increasingly evident. Regardless of the path, the important thing is to recognize that the simple fact of being conscious within the dream completely changes the experience. The dreamer ceases to be a passive spectator and becomes an active participant.

Research shows that about half the population has had at least one spontaneous lucid dream in their lifetime. This suggests that dream consciousness isn't a rare skill, but rather a natural extension of the human mind. However, the frequency of these dreams varies greatly from person to person. Some people have them regularly, while others only experience them occasionally. The good news is that, with practice and appropriate techniques, anyone can learn to induce lucid dreams more often.

The distinction between an ordinary dream and a lucid dream may seem clear in theory, but in practice, the line between the two states isn't always so defined.

There are times when a dreamer may have a vague notion that they're dreaming, but without the full clarity to act with intention. Other times, lucidity may last only a few seconds before the person gets lost in the dream narrative again.

The human brain is highly plastic, and training dream lucidity follows principles similar to developing any other mental skill. Just as we can train memory or mindfulness, we can train the mind to recognize patterns in dreams and awaken within them. To do this, it's essential to start paying more attention to your own dream activity. Keeping a dream journal, for example, is one of the first steps in the process. By recording dreams regularly, the brain begins to perceive that this content is relevant, naturally increasing the ability to remember and analyze nightly events.

Furthermore, understanding the difference between waking consciousness and dream consciousness helps us to see that the waking state can also be questioned. In our daily lives, we often go on autopilot, without being aware of the details around us. By training our perception of reality during wakefulness, this attention transfers to the dream world, facilitating dream lucidity.

One of the fundamental concepts in this process is the relationship between the conscious mind and the subconscious. In the waking state, the conscious mind dominates decision-making, but in the dream, the subconscious takes control, creating scenarios, characters, and events without us having direct influence over them. When we gain lucidity within a dream, we are essentially uniting these two states, bringing the clarity of the conscious to the territory of the unconscious. This integration can have profound effects, allowing the dreamer to explore their own psyche in a unique way.

Another interesting aspect of dream consciousness is that, contrary to what many people imagine, it's not just an esoteric or subjective phenomenon. Since the 1980s, scientific research has been demonstrating that lucid dreaming is a verifiable state. Studies conducted by researchers like Stephen LaBerge have proven that lucid dreamers can communicate with the outside world while they sleep, moving their eyes in a predetermined way within the dream. These experiments showed that dream lucidity is not just a subjective impression, but a measurable state of the brain.

Understanding how consciousness behaves in dreams also helps us overcome myths about the subject. Some people believe that it's possible to get "stuck" in a lucid dream or that the experience can be dangerous in some way, but these concerns have no real basis. The brain always returns to the waking state naturally, and lucidity within the dream doesn't alter the normal functioning of sleep.

Dream consciousness also presents varying degrees of depth. Sometimes, lucidity is light and fragmented, with the dreamer oscillating between clarity and confusion. Other times, lucidity is intense, with the individual perceiving every detail of the dream with extreme clarity. This variation depends on several factors, such as level of experience, emotional state, and sleep quality.

Training this skill requires patience, but the benefits are immense. From the moment the mind begins to recognize the dream state as a malleable and conscious space, the possibilities expand. The dream ceases to be a passive phenomenon and becomes an environment for exploration, learning, and discovery.

In the next steps of this journey, we'll see how the practice of lucidity can bring concrete benefits, from overcoming fears to enhancing creativity. The more we understand the nature of dream consciousness, the closer we get to the possibility of shaping dreams according to our will. And by mastering our dreams, we begin to realize that, in many ways, we can also shape our waking reality.

Chapter 3
The Benefits of Controlling Your Dreams

The mastery of dreams is not only fascinating, but it also profoundly transforms an individual's relationship with their own mind and emotions. The ability to awaken within a dream, to recognize the dream's illusory nature, and to consciously interact with it offers benefits that go far beyond mere curiosity. By controlling one's dreams, a person gains a new level of influence over their internal experiences, developing skills that can positively impact their waking life. From overcoming traumas and fears to enhancing creativity and emotional well-being, lucid dreaming reveals itself as a powerful tool for self-discovery and the expansion of consciousness.

One of the greatest benefits of lucid dreaming is its effectiveness in overcoming recurring nightmares. For many people, distressing dreams are sources of stress and anxiety, affecting sleep quality and, consequently, daily life. However, by becoming lucid within a nightmare, the dreamer can transform the threatening scenario, directly confront the fear, or even wake up at will. This process creates a sense of autonomy and resilience that extends beyond the dream world, helping the individual to deal with real-life challenges and anxieties with greater confidence and emotional control. Furthermore, the possibility of consciously interacting with the subconscious in a dream environment offers a unique means to process repressed emotions, promoting psychological healing in a natural and intuitive way.

Another fascinating aspect of lucid dreaming is its influence on the development of creativity and the enhancement of skills. The brain, when dreaming, operates without the limitations imposed by the logic and rationality of the waking state, allowing for the formulation of original ideas and innovative solutions to complex problems. Artists, scientists, and inventors frequently report moments of inspiration arising during sleep, and lucid dreaming potentiates this capacity by allowing the dreamer to deliberately explore scenarios, concepts, and unlimited possibilities. Moreover, research indicates that the brain activates neural patterns similar to those of real practice when rehearsing motor activities within dreams, making it possible to effectively train skills such as playing an instrument, practicing sports, or preparing presentations. By learning to consciously navigate the dream universe, the dreamer not only enjoys extraordinary experiences but also strengthens the mind, improves sleep quality, and gains a new perspective on their own reality.

One of the most immediate impacts of lucid dreaming is the ability to deal with nightmares. For many, recurring nightmares are a source of anguish, sleep deprivation, and anxiety. When someone learns to recognize that they are dreaming in the middle of a nightmare, the situation changes drastically. Instead of being a passive victim of dream events, the dreamer gains the autonomy to confront the threat, modify the scenario, or simply wake up. The feeling of being able to take control within the dream can be extremely liberating, gradually reducing the frequency of nightmares and promoting more peaceful sleep.

In addition to helping control nightmares, lucid dreams also have a direct impact on mental health. The simple act of perceiving and consciously interacting with one's own dream world develops a greater level of self-awareness. The subconscious mind expresses repressed emotions and internal conflicts through dreams, and when we are lucid, we have the opportunity to explore these contents with awareness. Many people report that their lucid dreams have become a kind of internal therapy, allowing them to confront fears, process emotions, and find answers to personal dilemmas.

Creativity is also amplified within a lucid dream. In the dream state, the rules of conventional logic are suspended, and the brain is able to create completely new scenarios, characters, and situations, without the limitations of linear thinking. Artists, writers, musicians, and inventors can use lucid dreaming as an experimental space where ideas flow freely. Many creators claim that innovative solutions to complex problems have arisen from moments of clarity within a dream. Salvador Dalí, for example, used dream states to visualize surreal images, while Nikola Tesla reported conducting mental experiments while sleeping. Lucid dreaming allows this creative exploration to become deliberate, providing an internal laboratory to test ideas, visualize concepts, and develop projects without the restrictions of the physical world.

Another fascinating benefit of dream awareness is the enhancement of motor skills. Research indicates that the brain, when simulating activities in a dream, activates neural patterns similar to those of real practice. This means that lucid dreamers can use this state to rehearse physical movements, such as playing an instrument, practicing sports, or even rehearsing a presentation. High-performance athletes already explore mental visualization techniques to improve their performance, and lucid dreaming takes this practice to an even deeper level.

Sleep quality can also improve with the practice of lucid dreaming. Some people fear that dream lucidity will interfere with rest, but, in reality, the opposite occurs. Having a more conscious relationship with sleep helps reduce insomnia and nighttime anxiety. When an individual learns to recognize patterns in their own sleep cycle and to interact positively with their dreams, they tend to sleep more peacefully and wake up more refreshed. In addition, the practice of lucid dreaming can increase the sense of control over one's own life, reducing stress and promoting a more balanced mindset.

The experience of consciously exploring the world of dreams can also be profoundly transformative on a philosophical and existential level. When someone realizes that they can modify the reality of a dream with their intention and expectation, they begin to question to what extent their own waking reality is as fixed as it seems. This questioning can lead to reflections on the nature of the mind, perception, and even identity. Many spiritual traditions use lucid dreaming as part of practices for expanding consciousness, exploring the intersection between waking and dream states to understand the true nature of reality.

Beyond individual benefits, there is also the social and cultural aspect of lucid dreaming. Throughout history, different traditions and philosophies have explored dreams as a way to obtain knowledge or connect with something greater. Today, science and spirituality are beginning to converge in this field, and lucid dreaming study groups are growing in communities around the world. Sharing experiences, exchanging techniques, and discussing discoveries with others interested in the subject can further strengthen the learning and practice of dream lucidity.

Upon realizing the breadth of benefits that lucid dreaming can provide, it becomes evident that this skill goes far beyond a simple pastime. It is a gateway to a new way of interacting with one's own mind, promoting personal growth, creativity, and well-being. And, throughout this journey, we will learn how to train this ability systematically, step by step, until it becomes a natural skill, available whenever the dreamer desires.

Chapter 4
Myths and Realities About Lucid Dreaming

Our understanding of lucid dreaming has often been clouded by popular misconceptions, sensationalized stories, and fictional portrayals. While the experience of awakening within a dream is profoundly transformative, there's nothing supernatural or dangerous about it. What it truly is, is a natural phenomenon of the human mind, accessible to anyone willing to train themselves. Separating the myths from the truths about lucid dreaming is essential to dispel unfounded fears and establish a solid foundation for its study and practice.

One of the most common misconceptions is the idea that a dream can cause real physical harm, such as death or irreversible trauma. This belief, often reinforced by fictional accounts, has no basis in science. The brain has natural protective mechanisms that ensure awakening when a dream experience becomes too intense. Similarly, the fear of becoming "trapped" in a lucid dream is unfounded, as the sleep cycle follows its normal course, naturally leading to awakening. Even in cases of "false awakenings," where the dreamer believes they have woken up within a new dream, consciousness eventually returns to the waking state without any harm.

Another recurring myth is the assumption that lucid dreams provide absolute control over the dream scenario and events. While it's possible to exert influence on the dream, the subconscious mind continues to play an active role in shaping the experience. The level of control varies from person to person and can be improved with practice. Furthermore, the belief that lucid dreaming is a skill exclusive to a select few is also mistaken. Anyone can develop this ability through specific techniques, becoming increasingly adept at recognizing and consciously interacting with their dreams. Separating fantasy from reality allows for a more objective and productive approach to the phenomenon, transforming lucid dreams into a practical tool for self-discovery, creativity, and mental well-being.

One of the most widespread myths is the idea that dying in a dream can cause real death. This belief likely arose from accounts of people waking up frightened from intense dreams, but there is no scientific evidence that a dream, no matter how vivid, can cause direct physical harm. What can occur is an intense physiological reaction – accelerated heartbeat, sweating, muscle tension – especially in nightmares, but this doesn't mean there's any real risk to health. The moment the brain perceives a state of extreme stress, it naturally awakens, ensuring the dreamer's safety.

Another common fear is the apprehension of getting stuck in a lucid dream, unable to wake up. This idea has been popularized by movies and fictional stories, but it has no basis in reality. Sleep follows natural cycles, and regardless of the experience within the dream, the body will always return to the waking state at the appropriate time. Even in situations where lucidity extends for a long period, there's a natural limit, as the brain doesn't maintain REM sleep indefinitely. In rare cases, a phenomenon known as "false awakening" may occur, where the person dreams they have woken up but is still within the dream. However, upon noticing the inconsistency of the environment, the dreamer quickly awakens for real.

Beyond unfounded fears, there are also exaggerations about the level of control that a lucid dream offers. Some people believe that, upon becoming lucid, they will immediately have absolute control over everything that happens in the dream, being able to alter scenarios and characters with a simple thought. While it is possible to modify elements of the dream, this doesn't always happen instantly or as expected. The subconscious mind still plays an active role in creating the dream environment, and many factors influence the ease of manipulation. In some cases, the dreamer themselves needs to train their ability to influence over time.

There are also those who associate lucid dreams with something supernatural, viewing them as mystical experiences involving parallel dimensions or communication with spirits. This interpretation varies according to personal beliefs, but from a scientific point of view, lucid dreams are natural processes of the brain, resulting from the activation of certain areas of the mind during REM sleep. The fact that they are vivid and intense experiences may give the impression that they go beyond the individual mind, but there's no proof that they involve anything beyond the dreamer's own psyche.

Another frequent myth is that only a few special people can have lucid dreams. The reality is that anyone with a functioning brain has the potential to develop them. While some people have spontaneous lucid dreams more frequently than others, this doesn't mean it's a restricted ability. Just like learning a language or playing an instrument, dream lucidity can be cultivated with practice and dedication. Specific techniques significantly increase the likelihood of becoming conscious within a dream, and over time, the experience becomes more accessible and natural.

There are also those who believe that lucid dreams can be harmful to mental health. This concern may stem from the idea that playing with the perception of reality within dreams can confuse the mind upon waking. However, studies don't indicate any association between lucid dreaming practice and psychological disorders. On the contrary, in many cases, lucid dreams are used as therapeutic tools to help people deal with trauma, fears, and recurring nightmares. The only caveat made by experts is that, like any intense mental activity, it's important to maintain a balance and ensure healthy sleep, without sacrificing the quality of rest to pursue lucidity at any cost.

Over the past few decades, science has dedicated itself to studying lucid dreams with rigorous methods. Experiments conducted by researchers like Stephen LaBerge have shown that lucid dreamers can communicate with the outside world while sleeping, using pre-arranged eye movements. These studies have helped to validate the existence of dream lucidity and to demystify the idea that it is something esoteric or imaginary. Advances in neuroimaging have also shown that when a person becomes conscious within a dream, there is an activation of the prefrontal areas of the brain, which differentiates this state from normal dreams.

In light of these facts, it becomes evident that lucid dreaming is not a dangerous phenomenon, nor a skill reserved for a few, nor a supernatural experience. It's a natural capacity of the human mind that can be trained and used in a productive way. By clarifying these myths, the path is clearer to explore the techniques and practices that will allow the dreamer to access this state with greater frequency and control. With the correct understanding, lucid dreaming ceases to be a mystery surrounded by fears and becomes a fascinating tool for exploring consciousness.

Chapter 5
Sleep and Dream Cycles

Sleep isn't a uniform state of rest; it's a complex and dynamic process that directly influences how we dream and our ability to achieve lucid dreams. Far from being merely a period of inactivity, sleep is structured into cycles that regulate everything from physical recovery to memory consolidation and the organization of emotional experiences. Each of these stages plays a fundamental role in the quality of our dreams, and understanding this structure allows us to use sleep strategically to promote dream lucidity.

The sleep cycle, which repeats several times throughout the night, is composed of different phases, divided between non-REM and REM sleep. During non-REM sleep, the body undergoes a progressive sequence of relaxation and recovery, ranging from the initial transition between wakefulness and sleep to the deepest stage, essential for the body's restoration. In this phase, brain activity decreases considerably, making dreams less frequent and fragmented. In contrast, REM sleep – an acronym for "rapid eye movement" – is when the brain becomes highly active, producing vivid and elaborate dreams. It's in this stage that lucid dreaming becomes most likely, as the mind operates in patterns similar to the waking state, but without the interference of external stimuli that limit perception during wakefulness.

Mastering sleep cycles allows you to optimize the timing and conditions for practicing lucid dreaming. The duration of REM sleep increases progressively throughout the night, making the last hours of rest ideal for achieving awareness within the dream. Techniques such as programmed awakening and briefly interrupting sleep before returning to sleep can significantly increase the chances of lucidity. In addition, healthy habits – such as maintaining regular sleep schedules, reducing artificial stimuli before bed, and recording dreams upon waking – strengthen the connection between the conscious mind and the dream world. By aligning knowledge about sleep cycles with appropriate techniques, the dreamer can transform the act of sleeping into a richer, more exploratory, and deeply revealing experience.

Sleep is composed of cycles of approximately 90 minutes, during which the brain passes through different phases. These phases can be divided into non-REM and REM sleep. Non-REM sleep, in turn, is subdivided into three stages. In the first, the transition between wakefulness and sleep occurs, a light state in which consciousness still fluctuates. In the second, the body relaxes more deeply, and brain activity decreases, preparing for the later phases. The third stage is deep sleep, essential for physical restoration, strengthening the immune system, and muscle recovery. During this phase, brain activity is minimal, and dreams are rare and fragmented.

The most important stage for lucid dreams is REM sleep. It is at this time that brain activity intensifies, reaching levels similar to those of wakefulness. The eyes move rapidly under the eyelids, the muscles become paralyzed to prevent the body from reproducing the movements of the dreams, and the mind enters a highly imaginative state. Most dreams occur at this stage, and it is here that lucidity becomes most likely. At the beginning of the night, periods of REM sleep are short, but as the cycles progress, they become longer and more frequent, with the longest occurring in the last hours before waking.

This pattern explains why some lucid dream induction techniques involve waking up in the middle of the night and going back to sleep at a strategic time. Interrupting sleep just before a REM period increases the chances of entering this stage consciously. In addition, getting enough sleep is essential, as those who have short or interrupted sleep end up missing the longer REM periods, significantly reducing the opportunities for lucid dreaming.

Sleep regulation also directly influences the ability to remember dreams. People who sleep little or have irregular sleep patterns tend to have difficulty recalling their dreams, which can be an obstacle to training lucid dreaming. Dream memory is strongest immediately upon awakening, especially if it occurs directly from a REM period. If a person gets up quickly and gets distracted by other activities, the memories of the dream dissipate within minutes. This is one of the reasons why keeping a dream journal is so important: by writing down experiences right after waking up, you strengthen the connection with the dream content and train the brain to pay more attention to dreams.

Sleep quality also affects the depth and clarity of lucid dreams. Fragmented sleep, with frequent interruptions, can make dreams confusing and less vivid. On the other hand, deep and restorative sleep favors rich and detailed dream experiences. Practices such as maintaining regular times for sleeping and waking, avoiding stimulants before bed, and creating a quiet environment in the bedroom help improve the quality of sleep and, consequently, the frequency of lucid dreams.

Another relevant factor is the effect of REM sleep deprivation. When a person spends a period sleeping little and then has the opportunity to rest adequately, the brain tends to compensate for the lost time with a "REM rebound," increasing the duration and intensity of this stage. This phenomenon can be used strategically to facilitate the induction of lucid dreams, although it is not recommended to deliberately compromise sleep health.

Understanding sleep cycles allows the practitioner of lucid dreaming to use this knowledge to their advantage. Knowing when dreams are most intense, how to improve recall, and how to create the ideal conditions for productive sleep are fundamental steps to accessing dream lucidity more consistently. Instead of simply waiting for a lucid dream to happen by chance, it is possible to structure sleep in order to increase the likelihood of these experiences, transforming the practice into something more predictable and controllable.

Chapter 6
How the Brain Creates Dreams

The human mind, even at rest, never ceases its tireless activity, interweaving memories, emotions, and scattered stimuli to create dream experiences that defy the logic of the waking world. Far from simply shutting down during sleep, the brain enters a state of intense neural reorganization, where different regions work in concert to produce scenarios and narratives that may seem disjointed, yet reflect deep processes of the psyche. The phase of sleep known as REM (Rapid Eye Movement) is one of the most active periods of this phenomenon, with electrical waves coursing through brain circuits, activating areas responsible for emotion, memory, and sensory perception. The result is a tapestry of images and situations that, although fleeting and ephemeral, can carry symbolic meanings, reinforce learning, and even offer unexpected insights into lived reality.

Throughout the night, the brain experiences sleep cycles that alternate between periods of greater and lesser activity, and it is precisely during moments of heightened neural excitement that dreams take on their most vivid form. The amygdala, the center of emotional processing, intensifies its activity, making dreams charged with intense feelings that can range from pleasure to fear, while the hippocampus, responsible for memory consolidation, reorganizes fragments of daily experience, inserting them into peculiar narratives. At the same time, the visual cortex simulates landscapes and scenarios that, despite being unreal, can be extremely detailed. However, the reduced activity in the prefrontal cortex, a structure linked to logical thinking and critical sense, causes the dreamer to accept absurdities as normal, transitioning without resistance between disconnected realities and impossible events. This delicate balance between reason and emotion shapes the architecture of dreams and explains why we often find ourselves immersed in fantastic stories without realizing their incoherence.

The exact function of dreams is still a mystery debated by neuroscience, but research indicates that they play a fundamental role in psychological regulation and in organizing lived experiences. By revisiting memories, the brain not only reinforces learning but also processes repressed emotions, offering a kind of mental rehearsal for dealing with future challenges. Some theories suggest that dreams allow the brain to test possibilities without real risks, while others suggest that they are an inevitable byproduct of intense neural activity during sleep. Whatever their purpose, understanding the mechanisms behind dream creation paves the way for the development of lucid dreaming, allowing the waking mind to consciously interact with this fascinating inner universe.

Most dreams occur during REM sleep, when the brain is highly active, similar to a waking state. One of the most active regions at this time is the amygdala, responsible for emotional processing. This explains why dreams are often intense, charged with feelings ranging from ecstasy to terror. At the same time, the hippocampus, a structure linked to memory, participates in the process, retrieving fragments of past experiences and incorporating them into the plot of dreams.

The visual cortex also comes into play, creating images and scenarios with an impressive level of realism. During dreams, this region behaves similarly to when we are awake, simulating visual perceptions with great detail. However, the prefrontal cortex, responsible for logical thinking and rational control, shows reduced activity, which explains why we accept absurd situations without question.

This imbalance between emotion and logic makes dreams highly plastic, mutable, and often illogical. Unexpected elements appear without warning, transitions occur without explanation, and the laws of physics can be completely distorted. However, when lucid dreaming occurs, parts of the prefrontal cortex become active again, allowing the dreamer to regain their critical capacity and realize that they are dreaming.

The way the brain organizes dreams is also related to memory consolidation. During sleep, information received throughout the day is processed, organized, and, in many cases, incorporated into dreams. This is why we often dream of situations we have recently experienced or of concerns that occupy our minds before sleep. This relationship between memory and dream can be explored in the training of lucidity, since conscious attention to dream patterns can help identify them when they occur.

Another fascinating aspect of the dream process is how the brain fills in information gaps. During dreams, when something doesn't make sense, the subconscious mind tends to create automatic justifications to maintain the narrative's coherence. This explains why a scene can change suddenly without causing surprise: the brain simply adjusts perception so that everything seems normal. This phenomenon can be used to the advantage of the lucid dream practitioner, as learning to question these moments of inconsistency is one of the keys to awakening within the dream.

The different theories about the function of dreams try to explain why the brain dedicates so much energy to these experiences during sleep. Some approaches suggest that dreams serve to process emotions and aid in psychological regulation, while others suggest that they may be a mental rehearsal mechanism, allowing the mind to test different responses to challenging situations without real risks. There is also the hypothesis that dreams are a byproduct of brain activity during sleep, without a specific purpose, but with side effects that influence our mental and creative state throughout the day.

Regardless of the exact function of dreams, understanding how the brain constructs them helps to realize that, far from being mere disconnected illusions, they are reflections of the mind's inner workings. When someone becomes lucid within a dream, they are essentially accessing this process consciously, intentionally navigating the creations of their own brain. This reinforces the idea that dreams, even in their apparent randomness, follow patterns and mechanisms that can be understood and explored.

As we progress in the development of lucid dreaming, this scientific understanding becomes a powerful ally. Knowing how dreams are formed allows the dreamer to observe them more closely, identify recurring elements, and, over time, learn to consciously interact with this process. The dream world, then, ceases to be an unknown territory and becomes an extension of one's own thought, a space where the mind can be explored in an intentional and transformative way.

Chapter 7
The Science of Lucid Dreaming

For a long time, lucid dreams were shrouded in mystery, considered rare and subjective phenomena, relegated to the realm of spirituality or folklore. However, scientific advances in recent decades have demonstrated that this experience is not only real but can also be investigated, documented, and even induced. Neuroscience and psychology have dedicated themselves to understanding the brain mechanisms behind oneiric lucidity, revealing that this hybrid state between sleep and wakefulness has concrete neurological foundations. Today, the study of lucid dreams is not limited to mere academic curiosity, but expands to therapeutic and cognitive applications, suggesting that awareness within the dream can be a powerful tool for self-discovery, overcoming trauma, and even improving motor and creative skills.

The first scientific evidence proving the existence of lucid dreaming emerged from groundbreaking experiments conducted in the 1970s. Researchers faced a fundamental challenge: how to prove that a dreamer was truly conscious within a dream, rather than simply reporting the experience upon waking? The answer came from the use of eye movements as a means of communication between the dreamer and the external world. During REM sleep, the phase in which the most vivid dreams occur, the eye muscles remain active, which allowed volunteers, previously trained, to perform specific patterns of eye movement within the dream. These signals were recorded by electrooculograms, providing the first objective proof that the dreamer was able to consciously perceive and interact with their own dream. This milestone paved the way for a new era of research, leading scientists to explore how the brain modulates the experience of oneiric lucidity.

With the advancement of neuroimaging techniques, it became possible to map what happens in the brain during a lucid dream. Studies show that, upon becoming lucid, the brain exhibits a distinct pattern of activation, combining characteristics of sleep and wakefulness. The dorsolateral prefrontal cortex, a region associated with self-reflection and critical thinking, shows a significant increase in activity, contrasting with normal dreams, in which this area remains less active. This phenomenon explains why, upon acquiring lucidity, the dreamer begins to question the logic of events and recognize that they are dreaming. Furthermore, research indicates that the practice of lucid dreaming can have positive impacts on emotional regulation, the reduction of recurring nightmares, and even cognitive development. These findings not only validate the experience of oneiric lucidity but also offer new perspectives on the functioning of consciousness and its interactions with the sleep state.

The first concrete scientific evidence emerged in the 1970s, when researchers began looking for objective ways to prove that a person could become conscious within their own dream. The problem was simple: how to prove that someone was truly lucid during REM sleep and not just reporting the experience upon waking? The answer came from innovative experiments that used eye movements as a means of communication between lucid dreamers and researchers.

The pioneer in this field was Keith Hearne, a British psychologist who, in 1975, conducted an experiment in which he asked a volunteer to move their eyes in a predetermined manner while lucid in a dream. Since the eye muscles do not suffer paralysis during REM sleep, this movement could be recorded by an electrooculogram, providing the first objective proof that oneiric consciousness was real.

Shortly after, Stephen LaBerge, a researcher at Stanford University, developed even more refined experiments. He created protocols for lucid dreamers to perform specific signals with their eyes during the dream, allowing researchers to observe in real time when lucidity occurred. LaBerge also developed methods to train people to induce lucid dreams deliberately, laying the groundwork for the popularization of this practice outside of laboratories.

With the advancement of technology, more sophisticated studies began to map what happens in the brain during a lucid dream. Using functional magnetic resonance imaging and electroencephalograms, scientists discovered that, when a person becomes lucid, certain areas of the brain associated with critical thinking and self-awareness, such as the dorsolateral prefrontal cortex, show an increase in activity. This contrasts with normal dreams, in which this region tends to be less active, explaining why we normally accept oneiric absurdities without question.

Another interesting finding is that, during lucid dreams, patterns of brain activity resemble a hybrid state between REM sleep and wakefulness. This means that, upon acquiring lucidity, the brain behaves in a unique way, mixing elements of the waking state with the immersion of the dream. This discovery reinforces the idea that oneiric consciousness is not just a subjective illusion, but a distinct and measurable state.

In addition to proving the existence of lucid dreams, science has also investigated their possible benefits. Studies indicate that people who train oneiric lucidity report a reduction in the frequency of nightmares, a greater sense of control over their emotions, and even improvements in sleep quality. There is also research exploring the use of lucid dreaming in the treatment of disorders such as post-traumatic stress, allowing patients to face traumatic memories in a safe environment within the dream.

Another line of research suggests that lucid dreams can be used to improve motor skills. Studies have shown that, by mentally practicing a movement within the dream, the same brain circuits activated during physical practice are stimulated. This raises the possibility that lucid dreamers can train in sports, rehearse presentations, or refine artistic techniques while they sleep, harnessing the power of mental simulation to improve performance in real life.

Studies on lucid dreaming continue to expand, with new discoveries emerging every year. Researchers are exploring ways to increase the frequency of oneiric lucidity, test different induction techniques, and better understand the neurological mechanisms behind this phenomenon. With the advancement of neuroimaging and artificial intelligence technologies, the future may bring even more insights into how dreams work and how we can use them intentionally.

What was once seen as a purely philosophical or spiritual theme has now become a legitimate field of study, where science and practice meet. The lucid dream is no longer just a subjective report, but a measurable, trainable phenomenon with promising applications. As knowledge advances, it becomes increasingly clear that the human mind has potential that is still little explored – and lucid dreams are one of the keys to accessing them.

Chapter 8
Dreams in History and Mythology

From the earliest civilizations to the present day, dreams have played a fundamental role in shaping myths, beliefs, and interpretations of human nature and the universe. Ancient peoples viewed dreams as divine manifestations, mystical revelations, or messages from beyond, attributing profound meanings to them that influenced political, religious, and social decisions. Before science unraveled the processes of sleep and brain activity, dreams were considered bridges between the earthly world and spiritual or supernatural dimensions. Thus, throughout history, each culture developed its own methods of dream interpretation, recording symbolisms and seeking ways to understand and use these experiences to guide daily life. This perspective on dreams not only shaped traditions and rituals but also influenced philosophies and religious systems that endure to this day.

The Sumerians, one of the oldest civilizations, recorded dreams on clay tablets over four thousand years ago, associating them with premonitions and communication with the gods. This tradition spread to the Babylonians and Egyptians, who developed extensive manuals of dream interpretation, in which each symbol had a specific meaning. In Ancient Egypt, specialized priests were tasked with deciphering the pharaohs' dreams, believing that such nocturnal visions could guide the destiny of the entire nation. The Greeks and Romans, in turn, incorporated dreams into their philosophies and religious practices. Plato and Aristotle reflected on their nature and function, while temples dedicated to the god Asclepius received pilgrims seeking healing through the incubation of sacred dreams. The Oracle of Delphi, one of the most influential institutions of the Hellenic world, also used altered states of consciousness, often associated with dreamlike visions, to provide enigmatic answers to those seeking guidance.

In Eastern and indigenous traditions, dreams took on an equally profound and transformative character. For Tibetan Buddhism, the practice of Dream Yoga teaches adepts to remain conscious during dreams as a way to achieve greater mastery over the mind and reality. Among indigenous peoples of the Americas, such as the shamans of various tribes, dreams were considered spiritual journeys, opportunities to receive teachings from ancestors and nature spirits. The concept of the "visionary dream" was widely valued, achieved through rituals, fasting, and meditation. Over the centuries, the view of dreams has oscillated between the mystical and the scientific. Freud revolutionized the understanding of dreams by suggesting that they were expressions of the unconscious and repressed desires, while Jung introduced the idea of archetypes and the collective unconscious, in a way, rescuing the connection between dreams and ancient myths. Today, although science has advanced in the study of dreams from a neuroscientific perspective, the fascination with their symbolism and impact on the human psyche remains, revealing that this ancient experience continues to play a crucial role in how humanity understands itself and the world around it.

In Sumerian civilization, one of the first in history, dreams were already being recorded on clay tablets more than four thousand years ago. Kings and priests believed that the gods sent warnings and instructions through dreams, influencing political and religious decisions. This view spread to other cultures of the Middle East, including the Babylonians and Egyptians, who developed sophisticated systems of dream interpretation. In Ancient Egypt, there was even a "Book of Dreams," a kind of manual that helped decipher the hidden meanings of nocturnal visions. Dreaming of calm waters, for example, was considered a good omen, while dreaming of wild animals could indicate imminent danger.

The Greeks and Romans inherited this tradition and expanded it with their own philosophical approach. For Aristotle, dreams were manifestations of human thought in a state of rest, although they could carry important insights. Plato, on the other hand, suggested that dreams revealed repressed desires, an idea that would echo centuries later in the studies of Sigmund Freud. But beyond philosophy, the Greco-Roman world also saw dreams as a means of communication with the gods. The temples of Asclepius, the god of healing, were used for the so-called "dream incubation," where the sick slept in sacred sanctuaries in the hope of receiving a divine vision that would indicate the cure for their ailments.

In the Judeo-Christian tradition, dreams appear as important elements in the Scriptures. Biblical figures such as Joseph in Egypt and Daniel in Babylon were known for their ability to interpret dreams and predict future events. In the accounts of the New Testament, Joseph, the father of Jesus, receives divine guidance in a dream to flee with his family and escape the persecution of King Herod. The belief in spiritual communication through dreams remained strong throughout the Middle Ages, influencing the culture and religiosity of the time.

Meanwhile, in the East, traditions such as Buddhism and Hinduism explored dreams in a different way. For yogis and spiritual masters, dreams were not only symbols or messages but also a state of consciousness to be mastered. The concept that the dream world could be as real as waking life led to the development of practices such as Tibetan Dream Yoga, which seeks to train the mind to remain lucid both in sleep and in death, preparing the practitioner for transitions between states of consciousness.

Among the indigenous peoples of America and shamans from various parts of the world, dreams were seen as journeys to the spiritual world. Many tribes believed that dreams allowed contact with ancestors, nature spirits, and spiritual guides. For some cultures, each individual had a "power dream," a vision that revealed their mission or protective animal. Specific rituals were performed to induce visionary dreams, including fasting, meditation, and the use of sacred herbs.

Throughout history, the view of dreams has oscillated between the sacred and the scientific. With the emergence of modern psychology, theorists like Freud and Jung brought new perspectives. Freud saw dreams as manifestations of the unconscious and repressed desires, while Jung saw them as a dialogue with the collective unconscious, full of universal archetypes. These ideas influenced the study of dreams in the West and helped shape the modern understanding of their role in the human psyche.

With the advancement of science, dreams began to be studied more objectively, but this did not diminish their enchantment. Today, we know that they are products of brain activity and that they can be influenced by physiological, psychological, and cultural factors. However, the interest in the meaning of dreams remains as strong as in antiquity. The search for answers continues, and the possibility of controlling them lucidly adds a new layer of fascination to this journey that has accompanied humanity since its earliest days.

Chapter 9
Dream Incubation in Ancient Cultures

The practice of shaping and influencing the content of dreams has been with humanity since its earliest days, reflecting an ancestral belief that the dream world could be a pathway to communication with higher powers, a tool for self-discovery, or a means to resolve complex issues of waking life. Before modern science began to investigate the mechanisms of dreams, numerous civilizations developed methods to induce specific dream experiences, aiming to obtain spiritual guidance, answers to personal dilemmas, or even physical and emotional healing. This process, known as dream incubation, was a widely respected ritual, involving practices such as fasting, meditation, the use of natural substances, and sleeping in sacred places, where it was believed that dreams would acquire a deeper meaning.

In Ancient Greece, dream incubation was taken to a sophisticated level, especially in the temples dedicated to Asclepius, the god of medicine. Pilgrims from various regions traveled to these sanctuaries to participate in rituals that prepared them for a night of sacred sleep. It was believed that, by sleeping in a consecrated environment after undergoing purifying baths, prayers, and offerings, the dreamer would receive in their dream a visit from Asclepius himself or his priests, who would transmit guidance for the cure of illnesses or the resolution of problems. Historical accounts indicate that many of these experiences were interpreted as true divine revelations, reinforcing the idea that dreams possessed a prophetic and transformative character. Similar practices were observed in Ancient Egypt, where pharaohs and priests sought messages from the gods through dreams, often sleeping on specific stones that, according to beliefs, amplified the spiritual connection.

Other traditions, such as Mesopotamian, medieval Islamic, and indigenous cultures around the world, also valued dream incubation as an essential tool for daily life and spiritual development. In Mesopotamia, records on clay tablets describe meticulous rituals followed by kings and priests to induce prophetic dreams, including restrictive diets and the recitation of specific prayers before sleep. In the medieval Islamic world, Sufis explored dreams as a direct channel of communication with the divine, employing techniques of meditation and repetition of sacred verses to induce visionary states. Among indigenous peoples, such as Native North Americans, the vision quest was a rite of passage in which the individual would isolate themselves in nature, often fasting, to receive in a dream revelations about their life purpose. Today, although science has unveiled physiological aspects of dreams, the ancient practices of incubation continue to influence modern techniques of dream induction, demonstrating that, throughout history, humanity has always sought ways to explore and understand this intriguing universe of the unconscious.

The ancient Greeks were one of the cultures that most explored this practice in a systematic way. In the temples of Asclepius, god of medicine and healing, pilgrims carefully prepared for a night of sacred sleep. Before sleeping, they performed purification rituals, including baths and fasting, as well as prayers and offerings to the god. During the night, they slept in a special area called the *abaton*, where it was believed that Asclepius or his priests could visit the dreamers in visions and offer healing advice. Upon awakening, participants reported their dreams to the priests, who interpreted them and prescribed treatments based on the messages received. Many accounts claim that people left these temples healed or with a new clarity about their condition.

In Ancient Egypt, dream incubation also played a fundamental role in religious and political life. Pharaohs and priests used practices similar to those of the Greeks to obtain divine revelations. In some temples, dreamers slept on "dream stones," believing that this practice increased the likelihood of receiving messages from the gods. The Egyptians also had a detailed system of dream interpretation, which linked certain symbols to specific meanings, influencing important decisions.

In Mesopotamia, where some of the first organized civilizations arose, dreams were considered direct messages from the gods. Cuneiform texts describe rituals to induce prophetic dreams, in which the practitioner had to follow a specific set of rules before sleeping, such as avoiding certain foods or reciting prayers. The Babylonians had priests specialized in dream interpretation, who helped kings and leaders make strategic decisions based on dream messages.

In the medieval Islamic world, dream incubation was widely practiced by mystics and Sufis, who believed that dreams were a means of communication between God and the faithful. Many sought answers to spiritual questions or important decisions through the "true vision," a dream that was distinguished from others by its clarity and emotional impact. Some Sufis developed techniques of meditation and recitation of sacred verses before sleep to increase the chance of having these experiences.

Indigenous traditions around the world also developed their own methods of dream incubation. Among Native North American peoples, for example, there was the concept of the vision quest, a ritual in which young people spent days isolated in nature, often fasting, to induce dreams that would reveal their life mission or bring messages from the spirits. In some South American tribes, the use of psychoactive plants was employed to intensify dreams and facilitate contact with spiritual guides.

What these different cultures had in common was the belief that dreams were not random events, but meaningful experiences that could be cultivated and explored. Although the explanations for dreams varied – from divine messages to encounters with spirits – the central idea that one could influence dream content persisted throughout history.

Today, with the advancement of science, we understand that the mind can indeed be trained to direct dreams. Techniques of suggestion before sleep, visualization of desired scenarios, and repetition of affirmations are modern versions of these ancient dream incubation practices. Although beliefs have changed, the essence of this quest remains the same: to use the world of dreams as a tool for learning, growth, and self-knowledge.

Chapter 10
Dreams in Eastern Spiritual Traditions

Eastern spiritual traditions have long viewed dreams as portals to deeper dimensions of consciousness, where the mind can transcend the limits of ordinary perception and access heightened states of understanding. Unlike the Western view, which for centuries regarded dreams as subjective manifestations or mere creations of the unconscious, in the East, they are seen as opportunities for learning and spiritual awakening. Cultures such as Tibetan Buddhism, Hinduism, Taoism, and Zen Buddhism have developed sophisticated practices to explore the dream world, considering it an extension of the spiritual journey. In these systems, the separation between wakefulness and dreaming is only apparent, as both are manifestations of the same fluid and impermanent reality. Those who learn to awaken within the dream acquire tools to also awaken to the true nature of existence.

Dream Yoga, practiced in Tibetan Buddhism and the Bön tradition, is one of the most elaborate approaches to training dream consciousness. For the masters of this tradition, recognizing the illusion within the dream is an exercise that prepares the practitioner to perceive the illusion of waking reality, dissolving the fixation on individual identity and worldly appearances. Specific techniques are taught to achieve this level of awareness, including reciting mantras before sleep, specific visualizations, and cultivating mindfulness throughout the day. The practitioner learns to constantly question their reality, creating the habit of testing whether they are dreaming, until this attitude naturally transfers to the dream state. By mastering this practice, they not only gain control over their dreams but also develop a more lucid and awakened mind in everyday life.

In Hinduism, similar practices are found in Yoga Nidra, known as "yogic sleep," which allows the practitioner to remain conscious while the body rests. This state is considered a bridge between deep sleep and meditation, allowing access to more subtle levels of the mind without losing awareness. In Taoism, dreams are understood as manifestations of the natural flow of existence, illustrated by philosophical reflections such as Zhuangzi's famous parable about the butterfly and the questioning of the nature of reality. In Zen Buddhism, the impermanence of dreams serves as a reminder of the transience of all things, reinforcing the need for detachment. These traditions share the central idea that dreams are not mere brain phenomena, but rather territories for spiritual exploration. The knowledge accumulated by these ancient schools remains relevant, offering anyone who wishes to explore dream consciousness a path to greater mental clarity, mindfulness, and understanding of their own mind.

One of the best-known traditions in this context is Dream Yoga, practiced in Tibetan Buddhism and the Bön tradition. For Tibetan masters, dreams are a reflection of the illusory nature of reality. If in the waking state people believe that the material world is solid and permanent, dreams show that everything can be shaped by the mind. According to these teachings, perceiving the illusion within the dream is training to perceive the illusion of life, leading to ultimate spiritual awakening.

Practitioners of Dream Yoga spend years developing the ability to maintain uninterrupted consciousness, both in sleep and wakefulness. Specific techniques are used to strengthen this lucidity, such as meditations before sleep, mantra recitation, and visualizations that prepare the mind to recognize the dream state. The goal is not only to have control over dreams but to use them as a tool to expand the perception of reality.

In Hinduism, there are similar practices associated with Yoga Nidra, also called "yogic sleep." In this tradition, sleep is not seen as a period of total unconsciousness, but as a state in which the mind can remain alert on more subtle levels. Masters of this practice teach that it is possible to reach a state of deep awareness without losing perception, accessing a space of pure observation where the practitioner can witness their own thoughts and emotions without becoming attached to them.

In Chinese Taoism, dreams also play an important role. Taoist philosophers, such as Zhuangzi, reflected on the nature of reality by questioning whether waking life was more real than a dream. One of his most famous stories tells how he once dreamed he was a butterfly. Upon awakening, he wondered: was he a man dreaming he was a butterfly, or a butterfly dreaming he was a man? This thought influenced generations of Taoist practitioners, who saw dreams as an extension of the natural flow of existence.

In Japan, within the Zen Buddhist tradition, dreams are considered manifestations of the mind and opportunities for contemplation. Zen monks use mindfulness techniques to bring lucidity to the dream world, often meditating on the impermanence of dreams as a reflection of the impermanence of life. Training the mind to question the reality of dreams reinforces the understanding that all experiences, both in sleep and wakefulness, are transient and should not be grasped rigidly.

What all these traditions have in common is the view that dreams are more than a neurological phenomenon. They are a field for exploring consciousness, a territory where the mind can be trained to perceive the truth beyond appearances. While modern science seeks to explain dreams through brain activity, Eastern spiritual traditions see them as a path to liberation.

Even for those who do not follow these philosophies, the teachings contained within them offer valuable lessons on how to view dreams in a deeper way. The practice of dream lucidity, so valued in these traditions, need not be limited to entertainment or mental experimentation. It can be a means of developing greater clarity, mindfulness, and a deeper connection with one's own mind. Just as Tibetan masters, yogis, and Zen monks explored the dream world to expand their consciousness, anyone can apply this knowledge to transform their relationship with sleep and reality.

Chapter 11
Shamanic and Indigenous Perspectives on Dreams

Indigenous cultures around the world place dreams at the very heart of the interaction between the material world and the spiritual realms. They see dreams not merely as reflections of the human mind, but as portals to deeper dimensions of existence. In shamanic traditions, dreams aren't interpreted as simple manifestations of the unconscious; they are vehicles for communication with ancestors, nature spirits, and higher forces that guide the paths of individuals and communities. This perspective stands in stark contrast to the predominant view of Western science, which often reduces dreams to neurological processes devoid of transcendental meaning.

For indigenous peoples, the dream experience transcends the limits of ordinary perception, providing valuable teachings, spiritual revelations, and even premonitions about future events. The dreamer, in this context, is not just a passive spectator, but a traveler who can consciously interact with these realities, extracting wisdom and purpose from them.

Among various indigenous groups, dreams are considered an integral part of the spiritual and social development of each individual, being used in initiation rituals and healing practices. The shamanic learning process, for example, often begins with visionary dreams, in which the apprentice receives instructions from spiritual beings or comes into contact with entities that guide them on their journey. This knowledge is not acquired through conventional study, but through direct experience in altered states of consciousness, where the soul breaks free from the constraints of wakefulness to explore invisible territories.

The vision quest, a ritual practiced by various tribes around the world, exemplifies this relationship between dreams and spirituality. During this practice, young people or future shamans isolate themselves in nature, subjecting themselves to fasting and meditation in the hope of receiving a revealing dream that will define their role within the community. These visions may present spiritual guides in the form of animals, symbols, or messages that are carefully interpreted by the elders of the tribe.

The importance of dreams transcends the individual sphere, influencing community decisions and establishing deep connections between human beings and the spiritual universe. Many indigenous societies share dreams among their members upon awakening, seeking to interpret their meanings collectively to guide their actions in everyday life. In some traditions, it is believed that certain individuals possess the special ability to dream for the community, accessing hidden information that can prevent disasters, reveal cures for diseases, or indicate the best paths for hunting and survival.

Furthermore, dreams are considered essential tools in maintaining spiritual balance, being used to identify energetic imbalances, resolve internal conflicts, and even confront dark forces that may be negatively influencing the life of a person or the entire tribe. This broad and respectful view of dreams reveals a holistic approach to reality, where the dream dimension is recognized as a legitimate space for learning and transformation, capable of connecting individuals to their ancestral roots and the invisible forces that shape the world.

Among the indigenous peoples of North America, for example, dreams play a fundamental role in rituals and social organization. Some tribes believe that everyone has a spirit guide that can manifest in dreams, providing teachings and protection. To identify these guides, young people transitioning to adulthood undertake the vision quest, a ritual of isolation in nature, usually accompanied by fasting and meditation. During this period, the individual is expected to receive a significant dream that reveals their life mission or brings them a power animal, a personal symbol of strength and wisdom.

Shamans, considered intermediaries between the spiritual world and the physical world, often use dreams as a means of communication with invisible forces. In many traditions, the training of a shaman begins with intense dream experiences, in which they receive instructions from spiritual entities or learn to consciously navigate through dreams. These spiritual guides may appear in the form of animals, ancestors, or mythological beings, bringing messages that are interpreted and applied to the life of the community.

In the tradition of Australian Aborigines, there is the concept of the Dreamtime, a mythical and timeless reality that serves as the foundation for the creation of the world. For Aborigines, dreams not only reflect the human mind but are also a continuous manifestation of this sacred time, where ancestors left teachings that can still be accessed by those who know how to interpret the signs. Dreamers are seen as spiritual travelers who can move between dimensions, bringing knowledge that helps guide their tribes.

In the Amazon, among tribes such as the Ashaninka and the Yanomami, dreams are considered direct revelations of the spirit of the forest. The shamans of these communities frequently use power plants, such as ayahuasca, to induce altered states of consciousness and expand the perception of dreams. In these states, it is believed that the soul can travel beyond the body, encountering nature spirits, healers, and beings from other planes. The visions obtained are shared with the tribe and can influence decisions about hunting, healing illnesses, and even conflicts between groups.

For many of these cultures, dreams are a form of learning as legitimate as waking experience. The knowledge acquired in a dream can be as valid as that obtained through direct observation, as it comes from a source that transcends the intellect. The dream world, in this context, is not a fleeting illusion, but a dimension of existence as real as everyday life.

Unlike the Western scientific view, which generally sees dreams as a neurological process without transcendent meaning, shamanic traditions treat them as fundamental events for understanding reality. This approach raises interesting questions about the nature of consciousness. If such diverse cultures claim that dreams can be used to access knowledge and transform life, there is something in these practices that deserves to be explored more deeply.

The connection between dreams and shamanic spirituality is also reflected in the way these traditions deal with nightmares. While in modern psychology nightmares are usually interpreted as reflections of internal fears or unresolved traumas, for shamans they can be manifestations of energetic imbalances or even attempts at communication from spirits or forces of nature. Instead of avoiding these dreams, the practitioner is encouraged to confront and understand them. Some tribes teach that a nightmare can be a test, a challenge to be overcome within the dream, allowing the dreamer to gain strength and wisdom.

Another notable aspect of the indigenous view of dreams is the role they play in community life. In many traditional societies, upon waking, members of the tribe share their dreams with others, seeking meanings and guidance for the day. In some African cultures, for example, there are morning meetings where the dreams of the previous night are discussed collectively. The same happens in some North American villages, where elders help interpret the dreams of the young and guide them on what to do with these messages.

Although modern science has moved away from these interpretations, there is something valuable in the way these cultures treat dreams: they respect them. Instead of dismissing them as mere creations of the unconscious, they see them as part of a great network of communication between the individual, their community, and the spiritual world. This attitude can teach much to those who wish to develop dream awareness, as it encourages a more attentive and respectful relationship with one's own dreams.

By studying these traditions, it becomes clear that the practice of seeking lucidity in dreams is not a recent invention, nor an isolated phenomenon. Humanity has always sought ways to consciously interact with the dream world, whether to seek knowledge or to explore territories beyond wakefulness. Shamans and indigenous cultures have been exploring this possibility for millennia, and their methods offer valuable clues on how we can deepen our own practice.

For those who wish to learn from these traditions, one of the first lessons is to pay more attention to dreams. Creating the habit of writing them down, reflecting on their meanings, and sharing them with others can help strengthen the connection with the dream world. Furthermore, the courage to face nightmares and the willingness to explore the symbols that arise in dreams can open doors to transformative discoveries.

The shamanic view reminds us that dreams are more than ephemeral images that disappear when we wake up. They are territories to be explored, messages to be deciphered, and perhaps an invitation to expand our understanding of reality itself. Just as the ancient indigenous masters navigated the world of dreams in search of answers, anyone can learn to do the same, using lucid dreaming as a means to travel between worlds and unravel the mysteries of their own mind.

Chapter 12
Lucid Dreaming in the Modern Era

Our understanding of lucid dreaming has evolved significantly over time, moving from the realm of esoteric and mystical beliefs to become a subject of scientific study and a tool for personal development. Today, this practice is no longer seen as an isolated phenomenon or restricted to spontaneous experiences, but rather as a trainable skill capable of providing benefits ranging from creative exploration to improved mental health. The advancement of neuroscience, coupled with a growing interest in altered states of consciousness, has brought new perspectives on lucid dreaming, allowing an increasing number of people to access and understand this fascinating aspect of the human mind. Lucid dreaming, therefore, not only broadens the perception of reality but also opens doors to self-discovery and the experimentation of possibilities that, in waking life, would be limited by physical laws.

From the late 19th century, when the first systematic accounts of lucid dreams began to emerge in the West, to the present day, the quest to understand and induce this phenomenon has mobilized scholars, practitioners, and enthusiasts around the world. The Dutch psychiatrist Frederik van Eeden was one of the first to describe in detail the experience of lucid dreaming, and from then on, research began to develop, albeit marginally. It was only with the advances in neuroscience and experimental psychology in the 20th century that the validity of lucid dreams became widely recognized. Experiments conducted by Stephen LaBerge at Stanford University, for example, scientifically demonstrated that it was possible to be conscious within a dream and even interact with the dream environment in a controlled manner. These findings not only legitimized the topic in academia but also enabled the development of accessible techniques so that anyone could experience lucidity in dreams.

The impact of this practice goes far beyond mere scientific curiosity. Over the years, lucid dreaming has been explored as a powerful tool for skill enhancement, overcoming trauma, and expanding creativity. Techniques developed by researchers and practitioners enable dreamers to learn to consciously interact with their own fears, confronting recurring nightmares and reframing traumatic experiences. In addition, athletes and artists have used lucid dreams as a space for mental training, where they can refine techniques and test new ideas without the limitations of the physical world. With the advancement of technology, devices and applications have been created to aid in the induction of lucid dreaming, making the experience more accessible and frequent. Popular culture has also played a crucial role in disseminating the topic, with films, books, and video games exploring the possibility of conscious manipulation of dreams, sparking public curiosity and encouraging new research. Today, the exploration of lucid dreaming is not just a field of study, but a constantly expanding phenomenon, uniting science, technology, and tradition in the quest to understand and transform the human mind.

The rediscovery of lucid dreaming in the modern West began in the late 19th and early 20th centuries, when psychiatrists and researchers of mental phenomena began to take an interest in the subject. The term "lucid dream" was coined in 1913 by the Dutch psychiatrist Frederik van Eeden, who documented his own experiences of lucid dreaming. He realized that, in certain dreams, he was fully aware that he was dreaming and could, in some cases, modify the events. This account caught the attention of other researchers, but for a long time, lucid dreams remained on the fringes of science, seen more as a curiosity than as a phenomenon worthy of systematic study.

In the 1970s and 1980s, everything began to change with the experiments conducted by Stephen LaBerge at Stanford University. Determined to scientifically prove that lucidity in dreams was real and verifiable, LaBerge developed a protocol in which lucid dreamers made specific eye signals while they were sleeping. As eye movements are not paralyzed during REM sleep, researchers were able to record these signals in real time, proving that lucid dreaming was not just a subjective account, but a measurable state of mind.

From these findings, LaBerge not only legitimized the phenomenon in academia, but also developed practical methods to induce lucid dreams systematically. He created the Mnemonic Induction of Lucid Dreams (MILD) technique, based on intention and repetition of mental commands before sleep, and published books that brought the practice to the general public. With this, lucid dreaming ceased to be a sporadic phenomenon and became a trainable skill, accessible to anyone willing to practice.

At the same time, interest in lucid dreaming was boosted by movements linked to spirituality and expanded consciousness. The book "The Art of Dreaming" by Carlos Castaneda brought the concept to a wider audience by describing shamanic teachings on dream consciousness. Although his work mixes fiction and reality, it helped popularize the idea that the dream world could be explored consciously, reinforcing interest in practices that lead to lucid dreaming.

With the arrival of the digital age, the study and practice of lucid dreaming began to expand even further. Online forums, lucid dreaming communities, and study groups began to form, allowing people around the world to share experiences, techniques, and discoveries. Access to scientific information also became easier, allowing a growing number of people to become interested in this phenomenon.

At the same time, technology began to play a crucial role in the induction and study of lucid dreams. Devices such as lucid dream masks, which emit light or sound signals during REM sleep to alert the dreamer that they are dreaming, were developed to facilitate the induction process. Mobile apps began to emerge, helping practitioners record and analyze their dreams, while neuroscience advanced in mapping the brain during lucid dreaming.

In addition to the experimental and technological aspects, lucid dreaming began to be explored in various areas, including psychology and medicine. Therapies based on lucid dreaming began to be used to treat recurring nightmares and sleep disorders. Patients with post-traumatic stress learned to consciously interact with their nightmares, reducing the emotional impact of traumatic memories. Athletes and artists discovered that they could mentally practice within lucid dreams, improving skills and exploring new forms of creativity.

Interest in the subject has grown so much that, today, universities and research centers are conducting studies on the effects and applications of lucid dreams. Scientists are investigating how this phenomenon can impact brain neuroplasticity, improve learning, and even offer insights into the nature of consciousness. Some research explores the possibility of using lucid dreaming to simulate and solve complex problems, taking advantage of the mental freedom that dreams provide.

Beyond academia, popular culture has also helped spread the concept of lucid dreaming. Films like "Inception" explored the idea of a dream world where people can manipulate reality, sparking public curiosity about the possibility of controlling their own dreams. Series, books, and video games began to address the topic, reflecting society's growing interest in alternative states of consciousness.

Lucid dreaming, which was once seen as a rare and poorly understood phenomenon, now occupies an increasingly large space in the field of mental exploration and human development. It not only proves the plasticity of the mind, but also offers a glimpse of the infinite possibilities that exist within consciousness. What was once knowledge restricted to a few is now available to anyone interested in exploring the world of dreams with full awareness.

The future of lucid dreaming studies looks promising. As science advances and new technologies emerge, more people will have access to methods for inducing and exploring this state. What was once a mystery is now becoming a tool for self-knowledge, creativity, and understanding the human mind. By uniting ancient and modern knowledge, tradition and innovation, lucid dreams continue to evolve as one of the most fascinating territories of human experience.

Chapter 13
Preparing for the Oneiric Journey

The preparation for your journey into the world of dreams begins long before you close your eyes to sleep. It involves creating the right environment, developing healthy habits, and cultivating a mindset conducive to lucid dreaming. The crucial first step is to foster a deeper relationship with your own dreams, recognizing their importance, and paying close attention to the details of each nightly experience. Often, the difficulty in achieving lucidity isn't about the brain's inability to awaken within a dream, but rather a lack of familiarity and engagement with one's own oneiric world.

Making a habit of recording your dreams in a journal upon waking is one of the most effective ways to strengthen this connection. It allows you to identify patterns, recurring themes, and signs that can serve as triggers for lucidity. The more you write and reflect on your dreams, the more your brain learns to value and remember these experiences, naturally increasing the frequency of oneiric awareness.

Beyond dream journaling, physical and mental preparation play a crucial role in the oneiric journey. Quality sleep is essential for any lucidity practice, as it's during the deeper stages of REM sleep that dreams become more vivid and conducive to conscious awakening. Creating an ideal sleep environment means minimizing external distractions, regulating room temperature, and avoiding exposure to artificial light before bed, especially the light emitted from electronic device screens.

Similarly, dietary habits also influence the dream experience. A balanced diet, with foods rich in tryptophan and vitamin B6, can enhance dream intensity and promote dream recall. Avoiding stimulants like caffeine and alcohol before bed contributes to a deeper and more restorative sleep, essential for achieving states of lucidity within dreams.

Mental preparation involves both setting intentions and managing the emotions associated with the oneiric experience. Repeating affirmations before sleep, such as "Tonight, I will be aware in my dreams," acts as a hypnotic suggestion that reinforces the expectation of lucidity. Visualization is also a powerful technique: imagining yourself within a lucid dream, experiencing sensations, and consciously interacting with the dream environment creates a mental conditioning that increases the likelihood of experiencing this state in practice.

Furthermore, it's essential to address any unconscious fears related to lucid dreaming, such as the fear of the unknown or loss of control. Cultivating an attitude of curiosity and exploration, understanding that lucid dreaming is a safe space for experimentation, helps to dispel insecurities and emotional blocks that might hinder the experience. With proper preparation, the oneiric journey becomes more accessible and rewarding, providing rich, transformative, and increasingly frequent experiences.

The environment where you sleep plays a crucial role in the quality of your sleep and, consequently, in your dream experience. A dark, quiet, and comfortable room promotes more stable sleep cycles, increasing the chances of fully reaching REM sleep. Avoiding strong artificial lights before bed, especially those emitted by cell phones and computers, helps regulate the production of melatonin, the hormone responsible for sleep. The temperature of the environment also influences rest, with a cool and airy space being recommended. Small adjustments to your resting place can make a significant difference in the depth of your dreams and the ease of achieving states of lucidity.

In addition to external conditions, mental preparation is also essential. Many people go to sleep carrying worries, scattered thoughts, and disorganized emotions, which can make dreams chaotic and difficult to remember. Creating a ritual before bed, such as meditation or relaxation techniques, helps calm the mind and direct your intention toward oneiric lucidity. Deep breathing and visualization practices before falling asleep can be especially helpful in establishing a more conscious connection with the dream world.

Another fundamental aspect is setting an intention. Throughout history, spiritual traditions and dream incubation practices have demonstrated that setting a clear intention before sleep can directly influence dream content. Mentally repeating phrases like

"Tonight, I will be conscious in my dream" or visualizing a specific scenario within the dream reinforces this programming, increasing the likelihood of awakening within the dream experience. Daily repetition of this practice strengthens the bond between waking consciousness and dream consciousness.

Regular and well-structured sleep is one of the main pillars for the practice of lucid dreaming. Creating a routine of fixed times for sleeping and waking stabilizes sleep cycles, ensuring that REM periods – where lucid dreams are most likely – occur predictably. People who sleep few hours a night or have irregular sleep patterns may have difficulty developing oneiric lucidity, as sleep instability interferes with the brain's ability to enter deep states of consciousness.

The relationship between diet and dreams also deserves attention. Some foods and substances can influence sleep quality and dream intensity. Avoiding caffeine, nicotine, and other stimulants in the hours before sleep can help maintain a deeper rest. There is evidence that certain foods rich in vitamin B6 can increase the vividness of dreams, as well as some supplements that stimulate brain activity during REM sleep. However, any experimentation with supplements should be done with caution and responsibility, always prioritizing natural and healthy sleep.

In addition to these physical and mental preparations, it is important to address the emotional and psychological aspects of lucid dreaming practice. Many people have unconscious fears about the idea of waking up inside their own dreams, fearing losing control or facing unknown experiences. This type of blockage can impede progress on the oneiric journey. One way to overcome this fear is to develop a mindset of curiosity and exploration, remembering that lucid dreaming is a safe environment where nothing can cause real harm.

Another important psychological aspect is patience. Developing lucidity in dreams is a gradual process, which requires consistency and dedication. Some people are able to have lucid dreams quickly, while others need weeks or months of practice before achieving satisfactory results. Avoiding frustration and maintaining a light and positive approach helps to maintain motivation along the way.

Self-knowledge plays an essential role in preparing for the oneiric journey. Each person has a unique relationship with dreams, and understanding one's own dream patterns can facilitate the induction of lucidity. Observing which types of dreams are most frequent, which emotions predominate, and which elements appear regularly can provide valuable clues to recognizing when you are dreaming.

The journey to oneiric lucidity begins long before you fall asleep. Creating a conducive environment, establishing a healthy sleep routine, preparing the mind with intention, and overcoming potential emotional blocks are fundamental steps for those who wish to explore the world of dreams consciously. By aligning these elements, the dreamer establishes a solid foundation for richer, more stable, and meaningful experiences, paving the way for true mastery of the oneiric universe.

Chapter 14
Keeping a Dream Journal

Regularly recording your dreams is a powerful exercise that strengthens the connection between your conscious mind and the dream world. It allows you to better understand your nighttime experiences and, consequently, increases your chances of achieving lucidity within your dreams. The practice of keeping a dream journal not only enhances dream recall but also helps you identify recurring patterns, latent emotions, and personal symbols that can serve as triggers for conscious awareness during sleep. When the brain is trained to give importance to dreams, it responds by intensifying its ability to remember, making dream images more vivid and detailed. In this way, the journal becomes a true map of your inner journey, providing you with a means to navigate the universe of dreams with greater clarity.

To get the most out of a dream journal, it's essential to establish a disciplined routine of recording your dreams immediately upon waking. In those first few moments after you wake up, dream memories are still fresh but tend to fade quickly if not captured. Staying still for a few moments, with your eyes closed, and focusing on retrieving fragments of the dream can help you rescue important details before they dissipate. Even if your initial recollections are vague or incomplete, jotting down keywords or loose images will help strengthen your dream memory. Over time, continued practice increases your recall ability, allowing you to remember not just one, but multiple dreams per night, including their sequences and transitions. Moreover, describing your dreams in rich detail – recording settings, sensations, dialogues, and emotions – enhances your perception of the dream experience and makes it easier to identify elements that repeat over time.

Another fundamental aspect of a dream journal is the analysis of accumulated entries. When you periodically review your notes, patterns begin to emerge: certain places, characters, or situations tend to recur, revealing dream signs that can be used as triggers for lucidity. Recognizing these patterns and training them in your waking mind increases the likelihood of realizing when you are dreaming, an essential step in developing dream consciousness. Furthermore, dream interpretation can offer valuable insights into your psyche, aiding in self-knowledge and understanding internal conflicts. Maintaining this habit not only enriches the lucid dreaming experience but also transforms the act of dreaming into a journey of continuous learning and exploration, where the mind becomes more receptive to the messages that emerge from the unconscious.

Many people believe they don't dream because they rarely remember anything upon waking. However, the truth is that everyone dreams several times a night, especially during REM sleep. The problem isn't the absence of dreams, but the difficulty in capturing them before they fade away. Just like a muscle that isn't used weakens, dream memory can be enhanced with practice and attention. The more an individual gets used to writing down what they remember, the more details begin to emerge, and the feeling of immersion in dreams intensifies.

The dream journal should always be beside your bed, ready to be accessed as soon as you wake up. The first rule upon waking is to avoid sudden movements and keep your eyes closed for a few moments, trying to recover any fragment of a dream before allowing your mind to be distracted by the stimuli of the environment. As soon as a memory emerges, even if it's vague or disjointed, it's essential to record it immediately. Keywords can be written down first, and then you can expand on the details as your memory becomes clearer.

The way you record your dreams also makes a difference. Writing narratively, describing the events as if they were a story, helps to strengthen the connection with the dream content. Details such as colors, emotions, physical sensations, and dialogues should be included whenever possible. Even fragmented or seemingly meaningless dreams should be noted, as patterns may emerge over time. In addition, including the date and a title for each dream can facilitate organization and later analysis.

Beyond writing, other forms of recording can be explored. Some people prefer to draw pictures of dream settings or characters, while others use audio recordings to capture memories more quickly before they fade. The important thing is to create a consistent habit, as regularity in recording strengthens dream memory and paves the way for lucidity.

Analyzing recorded dreams is another essential aspect of the practice. When you review your journal periodically, patterns begin to emerge. Certain places, people, or themes may appear frequently, indicating recurring elements of your psyche. These patterns are known as dream signs, elements that can serve as triggers for dream lucidity. When you recognize these signs within a dream, you are more likely to realize that you are dreaming.

In addition to identifying patterns, reflecting on dreams can reveal deep aspects of the unconscious mind. Repressed emotions, concerns, and desires can manifest symbolically in dreams, providing material for self-knowledge. Some people use their dream journal as a tool for introspection, seeking connections between dream themes and waking life events.

The practice of recording dreams also helps to make dreams more vivid. When the mind perceives that dream content is being valued, dreams tend to become more detailed and engaging. Dreamers who keep journals report an increase in the clarity of settings, the depth of interactions, and the intensity of emotions within dreams. This increase in vividness facilitates the transition to lucidity, because the more realistic a dream seems, the greater the chance that the dreamer will question its nature.

The dream journal is not just a passive record, but an active training tool for dream lucidity. It strengthens dream memory, reveals hidden patterns, expands awareness of the dream world, and creates a bridge between the waking state and the dream state. Over time, this habit becomes a natural part of the dreamer's routine, transforming the act of sleeping into a richer and more meaningful experience.

By committing to this practice, the dreamer establishes a solid foundation for the next steps of the journey. With a sharper dream memory and a well-documented repertoire of dreams, they will be better prepared to recognize when they are dreaming and, eventually, take control of their experience within the dream world.

Chapter 15
Improving Dream Recall

Dream recall is a skill that can be trained and honed with dedication and the right approach. It allows dreamers to access their oneiric experiences more clearly and use them as a foundation for achieving lucidity. While everyone dreams every night, many people struggle to remember these experiences because the brain doesn't automatically prioritize the retention of dream content. Therefore, to strengthen dream recall, it's necessary to adopt strategies that help capture and store dreams before they fade away. The first and most important step is to develop a clear intention to remember your dreams. This can be done through mental repetition before falling asleep, establishing a commitment to remember your dreams upon waking. This simple exercise of suggestion focuses the mind on the dream experience, increasing the likelihood that dreams will be retrieved more easily.

The way you wake up also directly influences your ability to retain dream memories. Ideally, avoid abrupt movements upon waking, as the rapid transition between sleep and wakefulness can completely erase dream memories. Remaining with your eyes closed for a few moments and trying to mentally relive the last sensations or images perceived before waking helps to recover fragments of dreams. If the memory seems vague, changing position in bed can stimulate different areas of memory and retrieve additional details. Furthermore, keeping a dream journal beside the bed and immediately recording any remembered fragment strengthens the habit of paying attention to dreams, training the mind to retain them for longer. Even if the initial notes are just loose words or disconnected images, over time, dream memory expands, allowing the recall of longer and more detailed sequences.

    Other factors also influence the ability to remember dreams, such as sleep quality and diet. Getting enough sleep to reach the deeper stages of REM sleep increases the intensity of dreams and their likelihood of being remembered. Having a regular sleep and wake schedule contributes to a stable sleep cycle, which improves dream recall. In addition, certain foods, such as those rich in vitamin B6 and tryptophan, can stimulate brain activity during sleep and enhance the vividness of dreams. By combining these habits with a mindful and curious attitude towards the dream world, dream recall becomes progressively clearer, providing a solid foundation for achieving and exploring lucidity with greater frequency and control.

    The human brain has the natural ability to dream every night, but remembering these events depends on specific factors. Upon waking, dreams tend to disappear quickly, often within minutes. This happens because the brain prioritizes waking information, and dreams, being experiences that have no direct connection with objective reality, are not efficiently stored in long-term memory. To overcome this limitation, some strategies can be adopted to capture fragments of dreams before they dissipate.

The first step to improving dream recall is to train yourself to wake up consciously. When opening your eyes in the morning, it's best to avoid any sudden movement and remain in the same position for a few moments. Moving your body quickly or starting to think about the day's tasks can interrupt the process of dream memory retrieval. Staying with your eyes closed and trying to remember what was happening before waking up helps to bring dream fragments to the surface. If nothing comes up immediately, changing position in bed can activate different memory states and recover memories that seemed lost.

Another factor that influences dream recall is sleep duration. REM sleep, where the most vivid dreams occur, becomes more frequent in the last hours of the night. Therefore, people who sleep little or have irregular sleep patterns tend to remember fewer dreams. Having a stable sleep routine and ensuring adequate rest time promotes increased dream activity and improves the ability to remember dreams upon waking.

Suggestion before sleep is an effective technique for reinforcing dream memory. Before falling asleep, mentally repeating phrases like "I will remember my dreams when I wake up" helps program the mind to value oneiric experiences. The repetition of these affirmations creates a clear intention, increasing the likelihood that the brain will retain and retrieve dream information upon waking. This technique is especially effective when combined with a dream journal, because by regularly recording dreams, the mind begins to understand that this content is relevant and worth remembering.

Waking up during the night can also be a useful strategy. As dreams occur in different cycles throughout the night, waking up at the right time can facilitate recall. Some people use alarm clocks set to times when they are more likely to be coming out of a REM period, which increases the chances of remembering dreams before they are erased by the transition to a deeper stage of sleep. Others prefer to wake up naturally during the night and record any dream fragment that comes to mind, even if it's just a feeling or a brief scene.

Diet and body biochemistry also play an important role in dream memory. Studies indicate that vitamin B6 can increase the vividness and recall of dreams, as it participates in the conversion of tryptophan to serotonin, a neurotransmitter involved in the regulation of sleep and cognitive processes. Foods rich in tryptophan, such as bananas, nuts, and dairy products, can contribute to deeper sleep and better dream memory. However, any dietary changes should be made in a balanced way, as excess stimulants or very heavy foods before bed can interfere with the quality of rest.

In addition to these strategies, developing an attitude of curiosity and attention to dreams makes the mind more sensitive to them. During the day, reflecting on past dreams, imagining how their unfolding would be, and sharing dream experiences with others strengthens the connection with the dream world. This habit creates a mental state conducive to recognizing and remembering dreams more easily.

Improving dream memory doesn't happen instantly, but with patience and practice, dreams begin to become more accessible. At first, only fragments may be remembered, but over time, recall becomes more detailed and complete. When this skill is well developed, the next step in the oneiric journey becomes more natural: noticing recurring patterns in dreams and using this information to achieve lucidity with greater frequency and control.

Chapter 16
Dream Signs and Personal Patterns

The human mind is a vast landscape where hidden patterns emerge during moments of rest, revealing profound aspects of the subconscious. Within the universe of dreams, certain elements repeat in peculiar ways, manifesting as recurring symbols that, when properly recognized, become keys to awakening oneiric consciousness. The identification of these signs doesn't occur randomly; on the contrary, it reflects the internal organization of each individual's experiences, memories, and emotions. Each person carries a unique repertoire of themes that permeate their dreams, acting as a reflection of their psyche and potentially serving as portals to the development of lucidity. This process of perceiving and analyzing dreams not only allows for greater mastery over oneiric experiences but also enables a deep dive into one's own essence, fostering self-discovery and the enhancement of consciousness.

Within this dynamic, the repetition of certain symbols or situations in dreams is not a random phenomenon, but rather a mechanism structured by the unconscious, which communicates through images and sensations. The mind uses familiar patterns to establish a connection between the waking state and the dream world, creating a guiding thread that can be traced by the attentive dreamer. Unfamiliar houses, recurring landscapes, mysterious figures, or even the experience of flying are just some of the manifestations that tend to repeat in dreams, being fundamental to the construction of a system of oneiric recognition. By perceiving these patterns, the individual begins to create a symbolic map of their own mind, identifying the elements that can serve as signs that they are dreaming. This mapping, when combined with practice and the development of specific techniques, becomes a powerful tool for achieving deeper states of lucidity and control within dreams.

The recognition of oneiric patterns not only enhances the ability to become conscious within the dream but also reveals emotional and psychological aspects that often remain hidden in the waking state. Recurring themes may be linked to past experiences, repressed emotions, or even unexpressed desires, functioning as a symbolic mirror of the unconscious mind. By recording and analyzing these patterns, it becomes possible to better understand the internal dynamics that influence both oneiric life and waking reality. The process of learning and familiarizing oneself with dream signs not only expands understanding of one's own inner universe but also paves the way for more vivid and controlled oneiric experiences, allowing the dreamer to interact intentionally with the dream world and explore its full potential.

Each person has a unique repertoire of recurring themes in their dreams. Some may frequently dream of flying, while others may repeatedly find themselves inside an unfamiliar house, meeting childhood friends, or facing specific challenges. These elements can manifest in various ways, but the underlying pattern remains, creating opportunities for the dreamer to realize that they are in a dream.

The first step in using dream signs to promote lucidity is to consciously identify them. Keeping a dream journal allows patterns to become evident over time. By reviewing the entries regularly, it becomes possible to notice recurring themes, frequent symbols, and situations that arise repeatedly. Noting these signs in an organized way, creating a list of potential triggers for lucidity, increases the chance of recognizing them at the moment they occur.

Dream signs can be classified into different categories. The first is *personal signs*, which include elements directly linked to the dreamer's history and emotions. It could be a place frequently visited in childhood, a significant object, or even a specific sensation that always manifests in the oneiric state. These signs are the most powerful, as they are deeply rooted in the individual's psyche and are more likely to appear frequently.

Another category is *impossible signs*, which include elements that could not occur in the waking world. Deceased people appearing in the dream, scenarios that defy physics, abrupt changes in the environment, or even the presence of extraordinary abilities, such as levitation and telekinesis, are clear indications that it is a dream. However, due to the inhibition of critical thinking during sleep, the dreamer usually accepts these situations without questioning them. By training the mind to recognize these anomalies, the possibility of awakening lucidity increases significantly.

There are also *subtle signs*, which are more difficult to perceive but still indicate that the oneiric reality is in operation. Sensations such as difficulty running, changes in the lighting of the environment, words that change when reread, and even the strange logic of dialogues can be valuable indicators that something is out of the ordinary. These details, although discreet, can serve as anchor points for awakening within the dream.

An effective strategy for strengthening the recognition of these signs is to set the intention before sleeping. Before falling asleep, the dreamer can mentally review the signs they have identified in their previous dreams and affirm that, if they encounter them again, they will know they are dreaming. This mental conditioning prepares the mind to react consciously when these elements arise in the oneiric state.

In addition to identifying recurring signs, developing a more questioning state of mind during wakefulness can increase sensitivity to perceiving inconsistencies in the dream world. Repeatedly asking oneself throughout the day if one is dreaming and observing details of waking reality helps to create a habit that can be carried over to the oneiric state. When this practice becomes part of everyday life, the mind begins to repeat this questioning in dreams as well, facilitating the awakening of lucidity.

Dream patterns not only aid in inducing lucidity but also reveal deep aspects of the unconscious mind. Certain recurring themes may be linked to unresolved emotions, past experiences, or repressed desires. Exploring these patterns consciously can offer valuable insights into one's own psyche, allowing for a greater understanding of oneself.

From the moment the dreamer learns to recognize the signs within the dream, the journey to oneiric control becomes more fluid and natural. Lucidity begins to occur more frequently and consistently, as the mind is already trained to identify the elements that indicate that one is dreaming. By enhancing this perception, the next step is to learn to actively test reality, consolidating oneiric consciousness and preparing to interact with dreams in a more intentional way.

Chapter 17
Reality Checks

The human mind operates within a delicate balance between wakefulness and sleep, processing information automatically and rarely questioning reality. During waking hours, we place complete trust in our sensory perceptions and the logic of everyday events, without needing constant tests to validate the authenticity of the world around us. However, within dreams, this blind faith persists, and the dreamer accepts even the most absurd situations as normal. The ability to discern between reality and dream requires the development of a more critical and questioning perspective, a habit that needs to be cultivated intentionally. This mental training involves challenging one's perceptions, incorporating small tests throughout the day to create an automatic reflex that will extend into dreams. Adopting this method strengthens the possibility of achieving lucid dreaming, allowing the individual to awaken within their own dream and interact with it consciously.

Reality checks work because they exploit the inconsistencies inherent in the dream world. In the oneiric environment, natural laws such as physics, spatial coherence, and visual stability are often altered without the dreamer noticing. By introducing small challenges into daily life that question these laws, the brain becomes more efficient at recognizing discrepancies when they occur during sleep. This process is based on repetition and conditioning: by performing tests regularly throughout the day, the mind internalizes the habit and carries it over to the oneiric state. However, this training requires more than just the mechanical repetition of the tests; a genuine state of doubt and careful observation is necessary. The act of sincerely asking oneself "Am I dreaming now?" should be accompanied by a detailed examination of the environment and a real attempt to find anomalies that might indicate a dream. When this level of attention is reached, the practice becomes much more effective and increases the frequency of moments of lucidity during dreams.

The systematic application of reality checks allows the dreamer to transform their own mind into an instrument of discernment. Small details that previously went unnoticed begin to stand out, and the perception of everyday experience deepens. This increase in awareness not only benefits lucid dreaming but also enriches the way waking reality is experienced. Questioning one's own existence and carefully observing the details of the world around strengthens the ability to stay present and conscious in all situations. In this way, reality checks become not only a tool for awakening in dreams but also a powerful exercise in mindfulness that positively impacts the quality of daily perception. As this habit solidifies, the barrier between the waking state and the oneiric state becomes thinner, and the transition to lucidity in dreams happens naturally, allowing for an increasingly deeper exploration of the mind and the dream universe.

Reality checks are simple yet extremely effective techniques. They consist of small experiments that challenge the rules of the waking world and, when applied within a dream, reveal its true nature. The secret lies in the constant repetition of these tests during the day, so that the habit automatically transfers to the oneiric state. The more the dreamer trains this practice, the greater the chance of performing it within the dream and realizing that they are dreaming.

One of the best-known tests involves counting the fingers on one's hand. In the real world, the fingers remain fixed, but within a dream, they often appear distorted, with altered numbers or strange shapes. Another test is to look at a digital clock or written text, look away, and then look again. In the dream, the numbers and letters often change illogically or become jumbled. Similarly, trying to pass a finger through the palm of the hand can be effective, as in the dream this action may be possible, revealing the oneiric nature of the experience.

Another powerful strategy is the breathing test. If the dreamer holds their nose with their fingers and tries to breathe, in the waking world the air will not pass, but within the dream, it is often possible to continue breathing normally. This anomaly serves as a clear sign that one is in a dream.

In addition to direct tests, mindfulness in waking life helps to increase sensitivity to unusual details. Often, what prevents lucidity in dreams is the fact that people spend their days on autopilot, without really observing the world around them. By cultivating mindfulness, questioning the environment, and paying attention to details, the dreamer develops a more critical eye that can be carried over to the oneiric state.

Creating reminders throughout the day to perform reality checks can help establish this habit. Setting specific times, such as when looking in the mirror, crossing a doorway, or hearing a specific sound, can condition the mind to associate these moments with checking reality. Another approach is to use an accessory, such as a ring or bracelet, that serves as a reminder to test whether you are dreaming.

The key to making these tests work is the seriousness with which they are performed. Many people perform the tests automatically, without really questioning reality, which reduces their effectiveness within the dream. For the test to be effective, it is necessary to genuinely doubt one's own state, asking oneself honestly: "Am I dreaming now?". This small act of doubt opens the possibility that, within the dream, the same question will arise, leading to lucidity.

Another important point is to perform more than one test whenever there is a suspicion that one is dreaming. Sometimes, a single test may fail, especially if the dreamer is very immersed in the dream narrative. Therefore, when performing a test, it is recommended to combine it with another, ensuring a more solid confirmation of reality.

With regular practice of reality checks and mindfulness in everyday life, the recognition of the oneiric state becomes increasingly natural. The mind begins to question its own existence spontaneously, and the moment of lucidity arises more frequently. This training creates the foundation for a more refined control of dreams, allowing the dreamer not only to realize that they are dreaming but also to interact consciously with the experience. With this habit well established, the next step will be to explore ways to direct dreams towards specific goals, further deepening mastery over the dream world.

Chapter 18
Dream Incubation and Intention

The human mind possesses a remarkable capacity to steer its dream experiences through intention and conscious focus. During waking hours, thoughts and emotions shape our perceptions and influence how the brain processes reality. This same principle applies to the world of dreams, where suggestions and desires formulated before sleep can significantly affect dream content. Dream incubation is a method that leverages this natural characteristic of the mind to guide nocturnal experiences, allowing the dreamer to set specific purposes for their dreams. Whether it's achieving lucidity, exploring particular scenarios, or finding answers to personal questions, incubation enables a higher degree of interaction with one's own subconscious. This practice transforms the act of dreaming into something deliberate and directed, strengthening the bond between consciousness and the dream world.

The incubation process begins in the period leading up to sleep, a time when the mind enters a state of heightened receptivity. The transition between wakefulness and sleep allows ideas and intentions to more easily infiltrate the subconscious, influencing the construction of dreams. For the technique to work effectively, it's essential to define a clear objective. The dreamer can visualize in detail what they wish to experience, mentally repeating affirmative phrases that reinforce their intention. For example, if the goal is to realize that they are dreaming, an effective suggestion might be: "Tonight, I will recognize that I am in a dream." This type of programmed affirmation directs the subconscious attention to identify elements that signal the dreamlike nature of the experience. Furthermore, consistent repetition of this practice strengthens the connection between desire and manifestation, making it more likely that the dreamer will achieve their goal upon falling asleep.

Beyond the mental formulation of intention, certain physical stimuli can enhance the effects of incubation. Writing the intention in a notebook or placing symbolic objects near the resting place reinforces the association between the waking world and the dream. Keeping a dream journal also aids in identifying recurring patterns and improving the technique, allowing for adjustments over time. The more familiar the dreamer is with their own dream themes, the more effective incubation will be. This practice not only increases the incidence of lucid dreams but also serves as a powerful means of exploring the subconscious mind. With dedication and patience, the ability to influence one's own dreams becomes a valuable tool for self-discovery, creativity, and personal development.

Incubation begins even before sleep, as it is during the transition between wakefulness and sleep that the mind becomes most receptive to suggestions. The key to a good outcome lies in formulating a clear purpose. Instead of simply hoping that a theme will appear in the dream, the dreamer needs to establish a firm and specific intention. This can be done by mentally repeating a phrase, visualizing a scene, or writing a small script for the desired dream. For example, if the goal is to recognize that you are dreaming, the suggestion might be something like "tonight, I will realize that I am dreaming." If the intention is to encounter a person or a place, one can visualize that experience repeatedly before falling asleep.

The use of physical reminders can also reinforce incubation. Writing down the desire on a piece of paper and reading it a few times before bed, or even drawing a symbol that represents the intention, helps to fix the idea in the subconscious. Some people prefer to place objects related to the dream theme near the bed, creating an association between the waking environment and the dream world. Small rituals like these strengthen the connection between daytime consciousness and the dream state.

Repetition is a crucial factor for the success of incubation. The more the dreamer reinforces the intention, the greater the chances that the brain will process this information during sleep. However, it's important to find a balance between determination and relaxation. Excessive expectation can generate anxiety, hindering the natural process of sleep. The ideal is to establish the intention firmly, but without rigidly clinging to the result, allowing the subconscious to act freely.

Beyond the content of the dream, incubation can also be used to facilitate lucidity. An effective approach is to link a previously identified dream sign to a reminder to question reality. If a dreamer frequently sees water in their dreams, for example, they can program their mind so that whenever they encounter water, they perform a reality check. This conscious-subconscious connection creates a trigger that can lead to spontaneous lucidity.

The effectiveness of incubation varies from person to person, but continuous practice increases its accuracy. Even if the initial results are not exact, any approximation to the desired theme already indicates that the mind is responding to the process. Reviewing the dream journal can help adjust the approach, identifying patterns and refining the suggestions until they become more effective.

Incubation can also be used to solve problems or seek creative insights. Many discoveries and inventions have been inspired by dreams, and the mind, when properly directed, can find unexpected solutions to everyday challenges. By setting an intention before sleep, such as finding an answer to a question or visualizing a project from a new perspective, the dreamer may awaken with fresh ideas and valuable insights.

This technique is not limited to practical matters; it can be applied to self-discovery and personal growth. Questions like "What do I need to understand about myself?" or "What is the next step in my development?" can be formulated before sleep, allowing the subconscious to bring symbolic and meaningful messages. These answers may not be obvious at first glance, but by analyzing the dreams carefully, patterns and meanings begin to emerge.

Dream incubation, when combined with other practices, such as dream journaling and reality checks, strengthens the connection between waking consciousness and dream consciousness. The more the dreamer learns to influence their dreams deliberately, the more naturally lucidity will become part of the dream experience. Gradually, control over dreams ceases to be something sporadic and becomes a refined skill, which can be applied not only to explore imaginary worlds but also to deepen the journey of self-discovery and creativity.

Chapter 19
Mnemonic Induction of Lucid Dreaming

The human mind possesses a remarkable capacity to forge connections between intention and memory, allowing us to recall specific information precisely when it's needed. This principle, known as prospective memory, is fundamental to the mnemonic induction of lucid dreams. Through deliberate mental programming, we can condition our brains to recognize the dream state *while* dreaming, thereby fostering lucidity. This approach leverages the mind's natural ability to retain and retrieve important information, strengthening the link between wakefulness and the dream world. When applied correctly, this technique not only increases the incidence of lucid dreams but also enhances dream recall and overall comprehension of the dream experience.

For mnemonic induction to be effective, it's crucial to establish a strong intention before falling asleep. The mind must be trained to identify recurring elements in dreams and, at the opportune moment, activate awareness within the dream state. The method involves reinforcing this intention through mental repetition and visualization. The dreamer should formulate direct, affirmative statements, such as, "The next time I'm dreaming, I will realize I'm in a dream," focusing on this thought with conviction. Furthermore, visualizing oneself within a previous dream, noticing something strange, and becoming lucid further strengthens this mental association. This type of practice creates an internal reflex that can be triggered at the right moment, leading to the awakening of consciousness within the dream.

Consistent repetition of this method, especially after brief awakenings during the night, significantly amplifies its effectiveness. Since REM sleep periods, during which the most vivid dreams occur, tend to intensify in the later hours of rest, practicing mnemonic induction upon returning to sleep strengthens the link between intention and dream experience. Patience and regularity are essential to consolidate this skill, making lucid dreams more frequent and natural. Over time, the mind becomes increasingly responsive to this process, allowing the dreamer to achieve a deeper level of control over their nocturnal experiences. This technique, when applied continuously, not only facilitates awakening within dreams but also broadens the understanding of the relationship between consciousness and the dream world, paving the way for even more advanced practices in exploring the mind.

This technique works best when applied immediately after awakening, whether in the middle of the night or in the morning, before going back to sleep. The first step is to recall the most recent dream, mentally reliving it with as much detail as possible. This process strengthens dream memory and creates a link between waking consciousness and the dream state. It's even better if the dream contains a characteristic sign that could indicate it was a dream. Identifying these elements helps reinforce critical awareness within subsequent dreams.

After recalling the dream, the next step is to set a clear intention. The dreamer should mentally repeat a phrase like, "The next time I'm dreaming, I will remember that I'm dreaming." This affirmation shouldn't be repeated automatically, but with full conviction, feeling the meaning behind the words. The stronger the intention, the greater the likelihood that it will manifest at the right moment.

In addition to mental repetition, it's helpful to visualize the exact moment of becoming lucid. The dreamer can imagine themselves within the previous dream, recognizing a strange detail and realizing they are dreaming. This visualization reinforces the connection between intention and the actual dream experience, training the mind to react in the desired way when the dream occurs again. This process should be repeated a few times until the feeling of expectation is well established.

Another important aspect of the MILD technique is maintaining focus on this intention until falling asleep. Often, what prevents lucidity is the mind quickly drifting to other thoughts before sleep. Staying focused on the purpose of remembering the dream and reinforcing the lucid intention while falling asleep significantly increases the technique's effectiveness. If distractions arise, simply return to the mental repetition and visualization, remaining engaged in the process.

The MILD technique becomes even more effective when combined with scheduled awakenings during the night. Since most lucid dreams occur in the later stages of REM sleep, waking up a few hours before the normal time and applying the technique before going back to sleep can significantly increase the chances of success. This method potentiates the intention, as the brain is already in a state conducive to continuing to process the suggestions implanted before sleep.

Patience and persistence are essential factors for the success of this practice. Some people achieve results quickly, while others need several attempts before experiencing a lucid dream. The important thing is not to give up if the first experiments don't result in immediate lucidity. Consistent repetition gradually strengthens the mind's response, making awakening within the dream increasingly natural.

Applying this technique not only increases the frequency of lucid dreams but also improves dream recall and connection to the dream world. The habit of reinforcing intentions before sleep makes the dreamer more aware of their own mind, helping to integrate the dream experience into waking life. As the practice becomes part of the routine, lucid dreams cease to be occasional events and begin to occur more regularly.

By mastering this approach, the dreamer moves closer to a more refined state of control over their dream experience. From this point, it becomes possible to explore even more advanced techniques, enhancing the ability to directly enter lucid dreams and prolong the duration of these experiences. Consistent practice of this technique translates into gradual and continuous progress, consolidating the ability to consciously awaken within dreams reliably and consistently.

Chapter 20
The WBTB Technique

Human sleep architecture follows well-defined patterns, in which the REM phase, responsible for the most intense and vivid dreams, becomes progressively longer as the night goes on. This knowledge allows us to apply specific techniques to optimize the occurrence of lucid dreams, making the conscious awakening within the dream a more predictable and controllable experience. The WBTB (Wake Back to Bed) technique is based on the idea of temporarily interrupting sleep and returning to it at the most opportune moment for lucidity, taking advantage of the fact that, after a brief awakening, the mind tends to maintain a higher level of activity when re-entering the dream state. This method, when applied correctly, significantly increases the chances of realizing that one is dreaming, providing a greater level of control and clarity within the dream.

The first step in effectively applying this technique is planning the exact moment of awakening. Since the sleep cycle occurs in phases of approximately 90 minutes, choosing the ideal time should take into account the natural progression of REM periods. On average, it's recommended to interrupt sleep between four and six hours after falling asleep, as it's during this interval that dreams become longer and more frequent. Upon waking, the dreamer should avoid sudden movements, remaining in a state of calm and introspection. Recalling the previous dream can be a great facilitator for lucidity, as mentally revisiting the recent experience strengthens the link between the waking and dream states. At this moment, the mind is particularly receptive to suggestion, making the repetition of affirmations such as "Next time I'm dreaming, I'll know I'm dreaming" a highly effective strategy.

The effectiveness of this technique can be enhanced by adjusting the time spent awake before going back to sleep. An interval of between 5 and 30 minutes is usually sufficient to keep the mind active without compromising the return to sleep. During this period, light activities such as rereading notes from previous dreams, practicing meditation, or simply reflecting on the goal of achieving lucidity help to reinforce the intention. However, it's essential to find a balance: if the time awake is too short, the mind may not be sufficiently prepared for lucidity; if it's excessive, it may be difficult to resume sleep and effectively access the REM phase. Consistent practice allows the dreamer to discover the ideal duration for their own biological rhythm, adjusting the technique in a personalized way. With consistent application of this method, lucid dreams become more frequent, providing not only greater mastery over the dream experience, but also a deeper understanding of the interconnection between consciousness and the world of dreams.

The first step to applying this technique is to determine a suitable time to wake up. As sleep cycles last approximately 90 minutes, a good starting point is to set an alarm to go off between four and six hours after falling asleep. This interval is ideal because it interrupts sleep during a phase when dreams are already more frequent and longer, but still allows you to go back to sleep without compromising rest.

Upon waking, it is essential not to move abruptly or get out of bed suddenly. Staying in a calm state helps preserve the remnants of the previous dream, facilitating the transition back to REM sleep. At this point, the dreamer can review the most recent dream and reinforce the intention to become lucid upon returning to sleep. Mentally repeating phrases like "Next time I'm dreaming, I'll realize I'm dreaming" is an effective way to program the mind for lucidity.

Staying awake for a short period before going back to sleep can make a big difference in the success of the technique. The ideal time varies between 5 and 30 minutes, depending on the person. During this interval, some light activities can help keep the mind engaged without fully waking it up. Reading about lucid dreaming, reviewing a dream journal, or even practicing a brief meditation are useful strategies for directing focus towards the goal of having a lucid dream.

However, it is crucial to find a balance. If the time awake is too short, the mind may not be alert enough to retain the intention of lucidity. If it is too long, it may be difficult to go back to sleep, compromising the quality of rest. The best approach is to test different durations and observe which works best for each individual.

When returning to bed, it's essential to maintain a relaxed attitude and allow sleep to occur naturally. Some people benefit from practicing visualizations, mentally recreating the setting of the previous dream and imagining themselves becoming lucid within it. This process strengthens the connection between consciousness and the dream state, making it more likely to awaken within the dream.

The effectiveness of this technique lies in the combination of a controlled awakening and a strategic return to sleep. This method increases the likelihood of entering directly into REM sleep with the mind still active, creating an ideal opportunity for lucidity. Many practitioners report that lucid dreams obtained in this way tend to be more vivid and lasting, as they occur at a stage of sleep where brain activity is already close to that of wakefulness.

One of the advantages of the WBTB technique is that it can be combined with other approaches to enhance the results. Mnemonic Induction of Lucid Dreams (MILD), for example, can be reinforced during the waking period, intensifying the intention to recognize the dream. Similarly, practicing reality checks immediately upon waking can help condition the mind to question the dream state throughout the night.

Patience is a key element for the success of this technique. Some people may need several attempts before finding the best balance between wakefulness and ease of falling back asleep. The important thing is to gradually adjust the process until it becomes natural.

When properly applied, this approach becomes a powerful tool for any lucid dreaming practitioner. The WBTB technique not only increases the frequency of lucidity, but also improves the quality of the experience, allowing the dreamer to explore the dream world with greater clarity and stability. By integrating it into the routine of practices, mastery of dreams becomes increasingly accessible, transforming nights into opportunities for conscious discovery and experimentation.

Chapter 21
Wake-Initiated Lucid Dreaming (WILD)

The conscious transition from wakefulness to the dream world represents a unique phenomenon in the exploration of consciousness, allowing the individual to transcend the boundaries between reality and imagination without losing lucidity. This journey begins with a deep understanding of the mechanisms of sleep and how the mind can be trained to remain alert while the body relaxes completely. Unlike spontaneous lucid dreams, where awareness of the dream experience occurs later, this technique aims to guide the dreamer directly into the dream world with full control from the outset.

By mastering this skill, it's possible to access a state where the mind becomes the architect of its own dream narrative, shaping scenarios, consciously interacting with characters, and even exploring possibilities impossible in the physical world. The success of this practice depends on a delicate balance between relaxation and attention, requiring the practitioner to understand the subtle signs that indicate the transition to sleep, without succumbing to the oblivion of wakefulness.

The path to this transition begins with mastering deep relaxation, an essential condition to allow the body to fall asleep without the mind completely shutting down. Creating a conducive environment is one of the first steps: a quiet, dark place, free from auditory or visual distractions, facilitates the induction of this state. Adjusting body posture also becomes a determining factor, since uncomfortable positions can lead to interruptions in the process. Beyond the physical environment, mental preparation plays a key role. Controlled breathing techniques, guided meditation, and visualizations are effective strategies to reduce mental agitation and facilitate entry into the transitional state. The more familiar the practitioner is with these techniques, the greater their ability to sustain consciousness on the threshold between wakefulness and sleep, avoiding both premature awakening and total loss of lucidity.

As the body surrenders to sleep, several peculiar sensations may arise, serving as indicators that the transition is underway. Hypnagogic phenomena, such as abstract images, disconnected sounds, and sensations of floating, become more perceptible at this stage. Instead of resisting these manifestations, the key to the continuity of the process lies in passive acceptance, allowing the mind to observe these events without becoming attached to them. It is at this point that the dreamer may experience sleep paralysis, a natural condition in which the body remains immobile while the mind is still awake. Far from being an obstacle, this state can become a gateway to lucid dreaming, provided that the practitioner understands its nature and learns to use it to their advantage. With patience and practice, the conscious crossing into the dream world becomes a refined skill, providing not only fascinating experiences but also greater self-awareness about states of consciousness and the malleability of the human mind.

The process begins with deep relaxation. The ideal sleeping position varies from person to person, but in general, a comfortable posture that avoids muscle tension is recommended. The environment should be quiet, dark, and free of distractions. Since this technique requires a high level of attention, it tends to be more effective when combined with a scheduled awakening, applying it shortly after a period of sleep, when the body is naturally predisposed to quickly return to the REM state.

The transition from wakefulness to dreaming can be challenging because the body needs to enter sleep without the mind losing its clarity. To facilitate this passage, it's helpful to focus attention on a single point, such as breathing or the mental repetition of a short phrase. Some people prefer to count slowly, while others focus on bodily sensations, observing the lightness of the limbs or the change in the breathing pattern as sleep approaches.

During this initial phase, it's common to experience hypnagogic phenomena, which are images, sounds, or bodily sensations that arise spontaneously in the transition between wakefulness and sleep. These manifestations can include flashes of light, distant voices, tactile impressions such as floating or tingling, and even auditory illusions, such as music or noises with no apparent source. Instead of reacting to these sensations, the dreamer should simply observe them passively, allowing them to unfold without becoming attached to any of them.

If the process is well conducted, these perceptions intensify until a dream scenario begins to form. The secret is to allow this construction to happen naturally, without trying to rush it. When the dream begins to take shape, the final transition occurs by entering this environment with full awareness. Some strategies to facilitate this entry include visualizing a specific scenario and imagining yourself walking through it, or simply letting yourself "sink" into the flow of hypnagogic images until the separation between wakefulness and the dream disappears.

One of the main challenges of this technique is to prevent mental excitement from waking the body before the dream is fully formed. Anxious thoughts or attempts to rush the process can activate consciousness to the point of preventing entry into sleep. Similarly, there is a risk of losing focus and simply falling asleep without maintaining lucidity. Finding the balance between relaxation and vigilance is the key to making the method work.

Another common obstacle is sleep paralysis, which can occur during this transition. This state, in which the awake mind perceives that the body has already entered muscle atonia, can be uncomfortable for those who are not prepared. Sensations such as chest pressure, inability to move, and even auditory or visual hallucinations may arise. However, understanding that sleep paralysis is a natural and harmless phenomenon allows the dreamer to use it as a springboard to directly enter a lucid dream, relaxing and allowing the dream state to develop.

Consistent practice of this technique progressively improves results. At first, it may take time to find the optimal level of relaxation and focus, but with experience, the process becomes more fluid. Some variations can be tested, such as lying in a different position than usual to prevent the body from falling asleep too quickly, or adjusting the wake time before applying it to maximize the chance of success.

By mastering this approach, the dreamer acquires an unprecedented level of control over their dream experience. Unlike techniques that depend on recognizing signs within the dream, this one allows consciousness to be present from the beginning, ensuring greater stability and prolongation of the experience. This ability to navigate between states of consciousness strengthens not only the practice of lucid dreaming but also the perception of one's own mind, creating a deeper connection between wakefulness and the universe of dreams.

Chapter 22
Other Induction Techniques and Tools

The quest for lucid dreaming can be enhanced through a variety of approaches that go beyond conventional techniques, allowing each individual to find the method best suited to their profile and cognitive particularities. The human mind is extremely adaptable, and different stimuli can be used to facilitate the transition to states of heightened awareness within dreams. This means that exploring a diverse range of strategies, from subtle adjustments in routine to the use of technology and supplements, can maximize the chances of achieving lucidity during sleep. Personalizing these techniques, taking into account factors such as sleep cycle, level of suggestibility, and even diet, becomes a differentiator for those who wish to delve deeper into the universe of lucid dreams with more consistency. The great challenge lies in understanding that there is no single universal formula: while some people find success through simple changes in habits, others require additional stimuli to condition the mind to recognize when it is dreaming.

Among the various alternative strategies, the incorporation of sensory triggers during sleep stands out as an effective method to stimulate self-awareness within the dream. Devices such as induction masks, which emit subtle light signals during the REM phase, and apps that play suggestive phrases throughout the night, can act as anchor points to awaken lucidity without interrupting rest. Furthermore, certain meditative and deep relaxation practices help strengthen the connection between the waking and dream states, allowing the mind to transition between these two worlds more easily. Training perception, through frequent reality checks during the day, can also significantly increase the chances of identifying inconsistencies in the dream environment and, consequently, activating awareness within it. Small adjustments, such as creating a detailed dream journal and using visual reminders in everyday life, reinforce the habit of questioning one's own reality, making this practice an automatic reflex that manifests in the dream state.

In addition to technological tools and mental exercises, there is also the biochemical factor that can be explored to enhance the experience of lucid dreams. Certain foods and natural supplements, such as galantamine and vitamin B6, have a direct influence on the quality and intensity of dreams, making them more vivid and memorable. Some substances act on the regulation of neurotransmitters involved in REM sleep, prolonging this stage and increasing the chances of lucidity. However, the use of any substance requires moderation and understanding of its effects on the body, as the response may vary from person to person. Therefore, the real difference in the improvement of dream awareness lies in the intelligent combination of different strategies, adjusted according to the reactions and results obtained. Careful experimentation and systematic observation are essential to identify the most effective methods, allowing each dreamer to develop a set of personalized tools to explore the vast and intriguing world of lucid dreams.

One interesting technique is called Dream-Initiated Lucid Dream (DILD), based on the common phenomenon of dreaming that you are waking up in your own room, believing that you have returned to wakefulness when, in fact, you are still sleeping. Often, people have multiple false awakenings in a single night, but end up accepting the illusion without questioning it. To take advantage of this natural mechanism, the idea is to remain still upon waking, keeping your eyes closed and avoiding any movement. If the awakening is a dream within another dream, this immobility allows the dreamer to slide directly into a new dream state with full awareness. Even when the awakening is real, adopting this strategy can facilitate entry into a new lucid dream soon after.

Another efficient method is the Finger-Induced Lucid Dream (FILD) technique, which involves tricking the body into falling asleep while the mind remains alert. The practice involves lying down comfortably and, as you begin to relax, lightly moving two fingers – usually the index and middle fingers – as if you were playing piano keys in an extremely subtle way. This movement should be repeated rhythmically, but without effort, just to maintain a minimum of mental activity. If executed well, this technique allows for a direct transition to lucid dreaming without the practitioner noticing the exact moment they fell asleep.

Another interesting method is Cycle Adjustment Technique (CAT), which deliberately changes the wake-up time on alternate days to train the brain to be more aware at certain times of sleep. For one or two weeks, the person gets used to waking up 90 minutes earlier than their normal time, creating an unconscious expectation of alertness during this period. After this adaptation phase, the technique is applied only on specific days, leaving the other days without early awakening. The brain, conditioned to the anticipation of wakefulness, can trigger states of lucidity on days when the alarm does not go off, increasing the frequency of lucid dreams without much effort.

In addition to behavioral techniques, some natural substances and supplements can influence the quality of dreams and the propensity for lucidity. Vitamin B6, for example, is associated with more vivid and detailed dreams, especially when consumed a few hours before bedtime. Studies suggest that this vitamin can increase dream recall and intensify their colors and narratives, making them easier to recognize as dreams. However, high doses should be used with caution, as excess can cause side effects, such as tingling in the limbs.

Another widely used supplement is galantamine, a substance that modulates neurotransmitters involved in memory and learning. This substance has shown potential for inducing lucid dreams when taken during the night, usually in combination with the wake-back-to-bed technique. By increasing brain activity during REM sleep, its effect can result in extremely vivid and realistic dreams, although some people report that it can cause mild discomfort or early awakening. Like any substance that affects brain activity, its use should be done with moderation and responsibility.

Technology has also advanced to assist lucid dreamers, offering devices designed to detect when a person is in REM sleep and emit subtle stimuli that help awaken awareness within the dream. Sleep masks equipped with eye movement sensors can flash soft lights or emit specific sounds at the exact moment the dream occurs. The principle is simple: the brain incorporates these stimuli into the dream, allowing the dreamer to perceive the external interference and become lucid. Smartphone apps with smart alarms and recordings of subliminal suggestions are also popular alternatives, helping to condition the mind to recognize when it is dreaming.

The choice of the ideal technique varies from person to person. Some approaches work better for certain individuals, while others require adjustments or combinations to achieve satisfactory results. The most important thing is to experiment with different methods and observe which ones are most effective for your own sleep and dream patterns. Keeping a dream journal to record progress and adjust strategies as needed can significantly accelerate the journey towards mastering dream awareness.

By expanding the repertoire of techniques and exploring new tools, the dreamer gains more control over their nocturnal experience and increases the chances of accessing states of lucidity more consistently. Each method brings its own perspective and challenge, but all contribute to the improvement of awareness within dreams. The more resources available, the greater the flexibility to adapt the practice to individual rhythm and needs, transforming each night into a real opportunity for conscious exploration of the dream world.

Chapter 23
The First Lucid Dreaming Experience

That first lucid dreaming experience marks a pivotal moment in the journey of anyone seeking to expand their consciousness during sleep. The discovery that it's possible to be awake within a dream, fully aware that everything around you is a creation of your own mind, unleashes a powerful mix of emotions, from initial euphoria to a sense of wonder and empowerment. This moment reveals the malleability of dream reality and throws open the doors to a universe where the laws of physics and logic can be bent to the dreamer's will. However, for this experience to be more than fleeting, it's crucial to understand how the mind reacts to the sudden realization of lucidity and to learn strategies for maintaining that state for longer periods. Like any new skill, stability within a lucid dream develops with practice, patience, and conscious experimentation.

The first major challenge is dealing with the excitement that accompanies the recognition of lucidity. Many dreamers report that, as soon as they realize they're dreaming, a surge of adrenaline courses through their body, causing them to wake up abruptly. This natural response occurs because the brain associates intense emotion with the waking state, interpreting the excitement as a signal to awaken. To overcome this obstacle, it's essential to remain calm and anchor yourself in the experience. Techniques like deep breathing, rubbing your hands together, or serenely observing your surroundings help to stabilize the dream. Interacting with the setting, touching objects, or exploring their textures reinforces the sensory connection and prevents the dream from dissolving quickly. The stability of lucidity depends, in large part, on the ability to balance excitement with serenity, allowing the mind to gradually acclimate to this new state of awareness.

Another essential aspect is developing methods to prolong the experience, preventing lucidity from fading or the dreamer from waking prematurely. Shifting your focus between different elements of the dream, moving within the environment, and using verbal commands like "increase clarity" are effective strategies for maintaining control of the experience. When the dream begins to fade, actions like spinning your body rapidly or pressing your hands against a surface can help re-anchor your mind within the dreamscape. Additionally, avoiding fixating your gaze on a single point for too long reduces the chances of the scene collapsing. The first lucid dreaming experience may be brief, but each attempt strengthens the ability to sustain consciousness within the dream, allowing episodes to become longer, more vivid, and more engaging over time. By recording every detail of this experience upon waking, the dreamer creates a deeper connection with their own oneiric mind, accelerating the learning process and refining their ability to explore the reality of dreams with greater mastery and fluidity.

Lucidity can arise in different ways for each person. Some dreamers notice that something in the environment doesn't make sense — an object changing shape, the presence of someone who has passed away, an absurd situation being treated as normal — and, upon questioning the logic of the dream, consciousness awakens. Others may achieve lucidity spontaneously, without apparent reason, simply "knowing" they are in a dream. For those who regularly apply techniques, the moment may come as confirmation that their efforts have paid off: a reality check that finally fails or the memory that they were trying to have a lucid dream.

The first challenge of the experience is maintaining emotional control. Excessive excitement can be a determining factor for an early awakening. Many dreamers report that, upon realizing they are dreaming, euphoria takes over, and this sudden increase in adrenaline causes them to wake up abruptly. To avoid this, it is essential to adopt a calm and focused posture. Instead of getting carried away by excitement, it is advisable to breathe deeply and mentally affirm that the dream is under control.

Another important aspect is the stabilization of the oneiric scene. The first lucid dreams tend to be unstable, with the scenery dissolving quickly or the senses feeling confused. An effective strategy to strengthen the experience is to interact with the dream environment. Touching objects, feeling their textures, rubbing your hands together, or even verbalizing commands like "clarity now" are techniques that help anchor the mind within the dream. Moving deliberately can also contribute to stability. Standing still can cause the dream to lose its sharpness, while walking, exploring the environment, and paying attention to visual and auditory details strengthens immersion.

Often, lucidity lasts only a few seconds before the dreamer awakens. This phenomenon occurs because the brain is not yet accustomed to sustaining this state for long periods. Continuous practice improves this ability, allowing lucid dreams to become increasingly longer and more detailed. To prolong the experience, it is important to avoid fixing your gaze on a single point for too long, as this can cause the dream to crumble. Shifting attention between different parts of the scenery helps keep the mind engaged and present within the dream environment.

When you notice that the dream is weakening, some techniques can be used to avoid waking up. Spinning your own body within the dream, rubbing your hands together, or even touching the ground can help restore the feeling of immersion. In some cases, when the dream seems about to end, it is possible to try to "jump" to another scene mentally, visualizing a new scene and allowing the flow of the dream to continue.

Another factor that can influence the duration of the lucid dream is the level of involvement with the dream narrative. Some people report that, upon becoming lucid, they immediately try to exert full control over the scenario, forcing sudden changes or trying to fly without any preparation. Although it is possible to control aspects of the dream, it is more effective to start with small interactions, such as testing gravity, observing details of the environment, or talking to dream characters. This gradual approach helps to consolidate the experience without overloading the mind with excessive expectations.

Regardless of the duration of the first lucid dream, the most important thing is to record it as soon as the dreamer awakens. Writing down every detail, from the sensations to the actions taken, strengthens the dream memory and prepares the mind to recognize patterns in future dreams. This record allows you to analyze what worked well, what challenges arose, and what techniques can be improved.

With continued practice, lucid dreams become more frequent and natural. The first contact with lucidity may seem brief and unstable, but each experience contributes to the improvement of the skill. Gradually, the dreamer learns to remain calm, to interact with the environment, and to prolong the duration of the dream. Mastery of dream consciousness does not happen overnight, but with each new attempt, the mind adapts and becomes better prepared to navigate with clarity through the vast universe of dreams.

Chapter 24
Staying Lucid

Maintaining lucidity within a dream requires a delicate balance of emotional control, sensory engagement, and effective stabilization strategies. Achieving dream awareness can be fleeting if the dreamer doesn't know how to sustain the experience, as excitement or a lack of adequate stimuli can lead to abrupt awakenings or the dissolving of the dreamscape. The mind, upon realizing it's dreaming, tends to react with increased neural activity, which can cause an involuntary interruption of sleep. To prevent this, it's essential to understand how to strengthen the connection with the dream world and prolong lucidity. This skill develops with practice and experimentation, and the more one applies specific stabilization techniques, the greater the ability to consciously navigate the dream without interruptions.

Active interaction with the dream environment is a cornerstone of maintaining lucidity. Touch, for example, plays a crucial role in reinforcing immersion in the dream. By rubbing your hands together, pressing your feet against the ground, or manipulating objects, the mind receives tactile signals that help anchor it to the experience. Exploring different textures and temperatures also contributes to prolonging conscious perception. Furthermore, moving within the dream is an effective way to prevent it from fading. Walking, touching walls, interacting with elements of the scenery, or even feeling the wind on your face as you run are ways to strengthen the connection with the dream world. When the dreamer becomes an active participant, rather than a mere observer, the stability of the dream increases significantly.

Another crucial strategy is controlling visual focus. Staring at a single point for too long can cause the scene to lose sharpness and crumble. To avoid this, it's advisable to constantly shift your focus between different elements of the environment, absorbing varied details and expanding your perception of the surrounding space. Additionally, verbal commands within the dream, such as "Clarity now" or "Remain lucid," can reinforce stability, as the brain responds well to direct suggestions. If the dream starts to lose consistency, techniques like spinning your body or rubbing your hands together help restore immersion and prevent a premature awakening. Maintaining a calm and confident attitude, without the fear of losing lucidity, is also essential for prolonging the experience. The more natural this process becomes, the longer and more detailed the lucid dreams will be, allowing the dreamer to explore this universe with increasing freedom and control.

One of the most effective ways to stay lucid within a dream is to actively interact with the environment. Touch is one of the most powerful sensations for reinforcing immersion in the dream world. Rubbing your hands together, touching objects and feeling their textures, pressing your feet against the ground, or even touching the walls around you are ways to anchor your consciousness within the experience. The more sensory stimuli are activated, the more solid the connection to the dream becomes.

Another factor that can affect dream stability is visual focus. Many people report that when they stare at a single point for too long, the scene begins to crumble or fade. To avoid this effect, it's recommended to move your eyes constantly, exploring the details of the environment and shifting your focus between different elements of the scenery. This practice keeps the brain engaged and reduces the chances of the dream suddenly disappearing.

In addition to physical interactions, verbal commands within the dream can help reinforce lucidity. Some people find that verbalizing affirmations like "Clarity now" or "Increase stability" strengthens the experience and prevents it from dissipating. The brain responds well to direct suggestions, and repeating simple commands can be enough to restore the sharpness of the dream and prolong its duration.

Controlling emotional excitement also plays an essential role in dream stabilization. The excitement of realizing lucidity is natural, but if not managed, it can cause the dreamer to wake up quickly. Taking deep breaths, staying calm, and acting deliberately within the dream help to balance the experience. Instead of trying to perform grandiose actions immediately, such as flying or changing the scenery, it's more effective to start with simple interactions and gradually increase the level of experimentation within the dream.

If the dream begins to lose stability, some techniques can be applied to restore it before it dissolves completely. Spinning your body within the dream, as if you were a top, is one of the best-known approaches. This movement creates a reset effect, often transporting the dreamer to a new scene while preserving lucidity. Another effective technique is to rub your hands together vigorously, as the tactile sensation stimulates the continuation of the experience.

Another interesting strategy to prolong the duration of the dream is to reinforce the intention to remain within it. In some cases, just consciously remembering that you want to continue dreaming can be enough to prevent a premature awakening. The fear of losing the dream can have the opposite effect, so it's important to cultivate a relaxed and confident mindset that the dream will continue as long as necessary.

The dream environment can also offer clues about its stability. Some people report that when the light begins to dim, the dream tends to crumble. In these cases, creating light sources within the dream itself, such as turning on a lamp or bringing the sun back into the sky, can help keep the scene vivid. Similarly, if the sound begins to fade or the environment seems unstable, focusing on details and actively interacting can restore the clarity of the experience.

By practicing these strategies, the dreamer develops greater control over their dream experiences and learns to sustain lucidity for longer periods. The more these techniques are applied, the more natural they become, allowing lucid dreams to evolve from brief moments to deep and enriching explorations. Mastering dream stabilization is a fundamental step for those who want not only to become lucid but also to navigate the dream world with freedom and consistency.

Chapter 25
Navigation and Control in the Oneiric Environment

Mastering navigation and control within a lucid dream represents a significant leap in the exploration of oneiric consciousness. Unlike waking reality, where physical laws impose concrete limitations, the dream universe responds directly to the dreamer's intentions and expectations. This means that any action can be amplified simply by believing it is possible. From locomotion to the complete transformation of the environment, every element of the dream can be shaped according to the individual's will, but this ability doesn't emerge instantly for everyone. To navigate fluidly and modify scenarios intentionally, a gradual learning process is necessary, in which experimentation and the strengthening of confidence play essential roles.

Locomotion within a dream can occur in various ways, and understanding these variations is one of the first steps to expanding control over the oneiric experience. Walking is the most intuitive method, but many dreamers report that the sensation of their steps can be unstable, as if they were treading on malleable or floating ground. For those who wish to overcome the barriers of traditional locomotion, alternatives such as levitation, gliding, and flight become fascinating possibilities. Flying, for example, is one of the most desired aspects of lucid dreaming, but it may require practice to be performed accurately. The key to successful flight lies in absolute confidence that it is possible. Insecurity or hesitation tends to manifest in the form of difficulties, such as unstable floating or unexpected falls. An effective method for gaining control over this ability is to start with light jumps, allowing the oneiric body to become familiar with the absence of gravity before attempting longer, directed flights.

Beyond movement, the ability to modify the surrounding environment is one of the most impressive aspects of lucid dreaming. Some experienced dreamers can change scenarios instantly with just a mental command, but for most people, the transition requires indirect strategies. Creating portals, opening doors expecting to find a different location, or using mirrors as a passage to other realities are approaches that help the mind accept changes in scenery more naturally. Similarly, manipulating objects within the dream becomes more fluid with practice. Testing the transformation of small elements, such as changing the color of an object or making an item disappear, strengthens the perception of control and prepares the dreamer for more complex changes. Constant experimentation expands the malleability of oneiric consciousness, allowing each experience to become richer and more personalized. As mastery over this universe grows, the dreamer discovers that there are no limits to what can be created, explored, or modified, making each lucid dream a unique journey of discovery and infinite possibilities.

The most basic way to get around within a dream is simply to walk, exploring the environment as if you were in real life. However, many lucid dreamers report that movement can feel strange at first. Gravity might seem different, steps might be lighter, or the terrain might change unexpectedly. For those who feel limited by conventional methods of locomotion, other options can be tested. Floating lightly, gliding over the ground as if in a low-gravity field, or even flying are common possibilities reported by experienced dreamers.

Flight, in particular, is one of the most desired experiences within lucid dreams. However, not everyone can achieve it on the first try. Some people report that, when trying to take off, they end up floating only a few inches before falling again. Others describe being able to fly, but in an unstable way, as if pulled by invisible forces. The secret to developing this skill lies in expectation and confidence. In the dream world, believing that something is possible often makes it a reality. If there are doubts or insecurity, the subconscious may respond hesitantly. An effective approach is to start with small jumps, gradually increasing altitude until you gain the confidence to fly with more control.

Beyond movement, another fascinating ability of lucid dreams is the capacity to alter the surrounding environment. Some dreamers find that, by wishing to be in a certain place, the scenery transforms instantly.

However, for many, this transition doesn't happen automatically. Creating changes in the dream may require a more indirect approach. Instead of trying to modify the scenery with a simple command, it may be more effective to use elements within the dream itself to facilitate the transition. Opening a door expecting to find a new environment on the other side, looking into a mirror and imagining that it will lead to another place, or even spinning around completely while visualizing a destination are strategies that often work well.

Manipulating objects within the dream also follows the rules of expectation. Most people find that they can pick up items and interact with them as in the physical world, but, upon realizing the illusory nature of the dream, it becomes possible to modify these objects at will. A piece of paper can transform into a flower, a stone can turn into a piece of chocolate, and a simple touch can make a wall melt as if it were liquid. The more the dreamer allows themselves to experiment and play with these possibilities, the more natural control over the environment becomes.

Dream characters also play an important role in this experience. Unlike the scenery, which can be molded without resistance, the individuals who appear in lucid dreams often act independently, sometimes surprising the dreamer with their responses and behaviors. Some people enjoy interacting with these characters, asking them about the meaning of the dream or seeking advice. While it's difficult to determine whether these responses come from the subconscious or are simply random constructions of the mind, many report receiving profound messages and unexpected insights from these interactions.

For those who wish to deepen their control over the oneiric environment, the key lies in experimentation and progressive training. Starting with small changes, like modifying the color of the sky or moving an object from a distance, can help build confidence before attempting more complex alterations, such as creating entire cities or visiting fictional locations. The more the mind gets used to the flexibility of lucid dreams, the easier it becomes to shape this reality according to one's will.

Exploring and modifying the dream world is one of the most exciting parts of the lucid dreaming experience. The freedom to fly, create impossible scenarios, and interact with characters from one's own subconscious offers infinite possibilities for learning and enjoyment. The more you practice, the more natural the feeling of being in control becomes, transforming each lucid dream into a unique and unforgettable adventure.

Chapter 26
Transforming Fears

Dreams represent a direct reflection of the psyche, where emotions, traumas, and deep-seated fears manifest in symbolic scenarios. Within this oneiric universe, nightmares take center stage, provoking intense and sometimes distressing reactions. However, the ability to become conscious within a dream, a phenomenon known as lucid dreaming, opens up the possibility of reframing these experiences. Instead of being mere disturbances, nightmares can transform into valuable opportunities for self-discovery and overcoming challenges. The mind, upon realizing it is dreaming, gains a new level of mastery over the narrative, allowing the dreamer to change their relationship with fear, confronting it in a conscious and transformative way.

This conscious approach enables a transition from passivity to control, modifying the emotional impact of the nightmare. The realization that the terror experienced within the dream does not represent a real threat is a crucial first step in breaking the cycle of fear. Recognizing this illusion creates a psychological distance, making the nightmare a less terrifying and more accessible experience for rational exploration.

Furthermore, this understanding strengthens the dreamer's self-confidence, as they begin to perceive the power they have over their own mental creations. Instead of being a victim of frightening scenarios, the individual becomes the protagonist of their experience, able to interact with the dream environment actively and intentionally.

With practice, the lucid dreamer learns that the elements of their nightmares, however dark they may seem, possess hidden meanings that can be deciphered and reframed. The act of directly facing a threatening figure, conversing with what once seemed terrifying, or transforming the dream environment are strategies that demonstrate the potential of this practice. Each nightmare ceases to be a simple manifestation of fear and becomes an invitation to discover unconscious aspects that, when understood, can generate significant changes both in the dream world and in waking life. In this way, nightmares not only lose their destructive power but also become portals to inner growth and the expansion of consciousness.

The first necessary shift in perspective is understanding that a nightmare, no matter how frightening it may seem, does not represent a real danger. When the dreamer gains lucidity in the midst of a terrifying scenario, the simple recognition that everything there is a mental creation already significantly reduces fear. Knowing that nothing can actually harm them creates an emotional distance, allowing the dreamer to move from the position of a passive victim to that of an observer or even the controller of the situation.

The natural instinct within a nightmare is to flee from the threat. However, in lucid dreams, this reaction can be replaced by a more conscious approach. Instead of running from a pursuer, stopping and facing it can reveal something surprising. Many people report that, upon confronting frightening figures within dreams, they change shape, transform into familiar people, or simply disappear. This simple act of confrontation dissolves the tension and can provide insights into what that image represents within the subconscious.

Another effective strategy is to engage in dialogue with the elements of the nightmare. Directly asking the pursuer or monster why it is there can result in unexpected answers, which often carry symbolic messages about repressed aspects of the dreamer's mind. Some accounts indicate that, upon interacting with these figures, they lose their aggressiveness and become allies within the dream.

In some situations, the ideal approach may be to transform the setting. If the nightmare environment is dark and threatening, the dreamer can try to bring light to the scene, imagine that the space is changing, or visualize a door opening to a safe place. This deliberate change in the environment helps to reinforce the sense of control and dissolves the emotional tension of the dream.

The technique of changing one's own form within the dream can also be used to confront nightmares in a creative way. If a monster seems threatening, the dreamer can transform into something even larger or develop superhuman abilities to neutralize the threat. Creating protective shields, flying away, or even absorbing the energy of the nightmare to convert it into something positive are approaches that demonstrate how consciousness within the dream allows for a new dynamic in the face of fear.

Some people who suffer from recurring nightmares find in lucid dreaming a powerful tool to deliberately rewrite these narratives. By recognizing a nightmare pattern, it is possible to program the mind to respond differently. If there is a recurring scenario, such as being chased by an unknown figure or being trapped in a threatening place, the dreamer can set the intention before sleep to react consciously the next time that nightmare occurs. This type of mental reconfiguration can completely transform the experience and reduce the frequency of nightmares over time.

Exploring fears within a lucid dream can also bring benefits to waking life. Overcoming a panic situation within a dream strengthens the sense of control and security in the waking state. Many dreamers report that, by managing to deal with nightmares lucidly, they have developed more courage to face everyday challenges and anxieties. This connection between the two worlds demonstrates how conscious work within dreams can positively reverberate in the dreamer's mind and behavior.

Transforming nightmares into opportunities for learning and growth is one of the most fascinating aspects of lucid dreaming. When fear is no longer seen as insurmountable and begins to be understood as an aspect of one's own mind that can be explored and reframed, the dreamer assumes a new level of control over their dream experience. With practice and persistence, nightmares can cease to be terrifying events and become portals to self-discovery, courage, and the expansion of consciousness.

Chapter 27
Healing and Personal Growth

The human mind carries within it a vast territory of memories, emotions, and beliefs that shape our daily experience, often unconsciously. Lucid dreams, by offering direct access to this inner universe, become a powerful tool for promoting emotional healing and personal growth. By becoming conscious within the dream, the individual gains the ability to interact with their own psychic contents, understand limiting thought patterns, and reframe past experiences. This expanded state of perception allows for the exploration of deep emotional issues, fostering a process of self-discovery that can positively impact waking life.

Within a lucid dream, the mind reveals hidden aspects of the self, often through symbols and metaphors that express internal conflicts. The dreamer, upon realizing their lucidity, can use this space to dialogue with these images, understanding their meanings and unlocking repressed emotions. Instead of merely witnessing a dream unfold, the person becomes an active participant, able to question dream characters, modify scenarios, or relive situations from a new perspective. This process of internal exploration allows for a deeper understanding of traumas, insecurities, and emotional challenges, paving the way for overcoming them and achieving personal transformation.

Beyond emotional healing, lucid dreams also strengthen resilience and self-confidence. The simple act of realizing that one can interact with and alter events within the dream creates a sense of empowerment that extends into waking life. Situations that once seemed insurmountable gain new possibilities for coping, fears are dissolved, and the dreamer begins to see their reality with greater clarity and control. Thus, lucid dreams not only reveal internal aspects of the mind, but also provide practical tools to deal with challenges, strengthen self-esteem, and expand consciousness towards a state of greater balance and well-being.

One of the most effective ways to use lucid dreams for emotional healing is to connect with repressed emotions. Often, issues that we cannot fully process in the waking state emerge in dreams in the form of symbols, scenarios, or characters. Becoming lucid in the midst of these experiences allows us to interact directly with these elements and seek understanding. If a dream brings a persistent feeling of fear, sadness, or anger, instead of avoiding it, the dreamer can ask the dream itself what that emotion represents and allow their mind to provide spontaneous answers. This approach can reveal hidden connections between past events and unresolved feelings, facilitating the integration and processing of these emotions.

Encounters with past versions of oneself are another common phenomenon in lucid dreams focused on self-discovery. Some people report meeting their inner child, being able to converse with and offer affection and security to this part of the psyche that still holds traumas or insecurities. Others experience dreams where they encounter future versions of themselves, receiving advice or glimpsing possible paths for their personal journey. These interactions can have a profound impact on how the dreamer perceives themselves and their own life trajectory.

In addition to emotional work, lucid dreams can be used to overcome fears and phobias. Within the dream, it is possible to simulate situations that cause anxiety in waking life, but in a controlled and safe way. If someone is afraid of public speaking, for example, they can create a scenario where they practice a speech in front of an imaginary audience. If the fear is of heights, they can experience standing on top of a building within the dream and realize that nothing bad happens. The brain processes these experiences in a similar way to real-life experiences, which means that overcoming a fear within a dream can result in a reduction of anxiety related to it in the waking state.

Another valuable aspect of lucid dreams for personal growth is the possibility of receiving insights and answers to internal dilemmas. Before sleeping, the dreamer can set the intention to find a solution to a specific problem. Within the dream, upon becoming lucid, they can ask questions directly to the dream itself or to dream characters, expecting the answers to emerge symbolically or directly. Many people report that dreams provide creative and unexpected solutions to issues that seemed unsolvable in waking life.

Physical healing through dreams is also a topic explored by many practitioners and researchers. Although science is still studying the effects of this practice, there are reports of people who use lucid dreams to visualize the regeneration of areas of the body affected by illness or injury, feeling real relief upon awakening. The mind has a strong influence on the body, and the visualization of healing within the dream can stimulate internal processes that aid in physical well-being.

The practice of lucid dreaming as a tool for personal growth is also related to strengthening self-esteem and a sense of empowerment. The simple act of realizing that one has control over one's own reality within the dream can increase confidence and the feeling of autonomy in waking life. By consciously dealing with challenges in the dream world, the dreamer develops a more resilient and adaptable mindset to face real difficulties.

Integrating the experiences of lucid dreams into daily waking life enhances the benefits of this practice. Keeping a dream journal and reflecting on recurring themes allows one to identify internal patterns and work on conscious changes. The lessons learned in the dream state can be applied in real life, whether in the form of new habits, changes in perspective, or decisions more aligned with one's true self.

The journey within dreams is, essentially, a journey into oneself. When approached with purpose and intention, this experience becomes a portal to emotional healing, the expansion of consciousness, and personal growth. Lucid dreams offer the unique opportunity to explore the mind in its purest form, without external filters or limitations, providing discoveries that can profoundly transform the way the dreamer lives and understands their own existence.

Chapter 28
Creativity and Problem-Solving

The human mind operates in extraordinary ways when freed from the shackles of conventional logic, and lucid dreaming represents one of the most direct pathways to this boundless potential. In the dream state, the constraints imposed by linear thinking dissolve, allowing innovative ideas to flourish without the typical blockages of wakefulness. This unique environment provides fertile ground for experimentation, where abstract concepts can materialize, complex problems can be approached from unexpected angles, and creativity can expand in unprecedented ways. By awakening within the dream, the individual gains not only awareness of their experience but also the ability to explore it intentionally, transforming the dream world into a true laboratory of invention and discovery.

Interacting with this limitless mental space enables a form of learning and creation that transcends traditional methods. Writers can visualize their stories unfolding in real-time, engaging in dialogue with characters and exploring settings that emerge spontaneously. Musicians can hear original melodies created by their own subconscious minds, while visual artists can experiment with impossible compositions, exploring colors and forms beyond what they could conceive of in the waking state. Even scientists and inventors can benefit from this creative environment, where abstract concepts become tangible and problem-solving occurs intuitively, connecting information in unconventional ways. The brain, operating without restrictions, allows for the emergence of ideas that might be unattainable through traditional logical analysis.

Beyond stimulating creativity, lucid dreams enable the enhancement of practical skills through mental simulation. Science has shown that intense visualization can strengthen neural connections in a manner similar to actual practice. This means an athlete can train specific movements, a speaker can rehearse speeches, and even a student can deepen their understanding of a complex concept. The mind, perceiving the dream experience as real, processes these exercises as legitimate learning, making this a powerful tool for both cognitive development and overcoming practical challenges. Thus, lucid dreams reveal themselves not only as a space for entertainment or personal exploration but also as a valuable resource for unlocking new levels of creativity, solving problems, and expanding the frontiers of human thought.

The creation of scenarios, characters, and narratives within the dream occurs effortlessly, as the subconscious mind is capable of constructing images and stories in real-time. For a writer or screenwriter, this can mean the opportunity to explore scenes and dialogues even before putting them on paper. A musician can hear original compositions created by their own brain and even try to reproduce them upon waking. A painter or designer can visualize patterns, shapes, and colors never before imagined, using the dream as a space for limitless artistic experimentation.

Creativity in lucid dreams is not limited to the arts; it also extends to solving practical problems. Issues that seem insurmountable in waking life can find unexpected answers within the dream world. Before falling asleep, the dreamer can set the intention to solve a specific problem, formulating a question or mental challenge. In the lucid state, they can then seek the answer directly, asking for help from dream characters or exploring the dream environment for symbolic clues. Often, solutions emerge intuitively, without the need for linear reasoning, as the brain operates in a more free and associative manner.

Skill training also becomes an intriguing possibility within lucid dreams. Studies indicate that mental practice of physical or intellectual activities can strengthen neural connections similar to those formed during actual practice. This means that an athlete can refine their movements within the dream, a musician can rehearse a complex piece, and even someone who wants to develop social skills can practice interactions and speeches within the dream environment. The mind does not completely distinguish between imagined practice and real practice, making this strategy a valuable tool for learning and personal development.

Beyond skill enhancement, lucid dreams can be used to experience new perspectives and expand creativity in unexpected ways. An interesting exercise is to change form within the dream, assuming the point of view of an animal, an object, or even another human being. This shift in perspective can generate profound insights into empathy, imagination, and understanding the world from angles different from the usual ones.

Another effective method for stimulating creativity within a lucid dream is to challenge the rules of the dream environment. Playing with the laws of physics, creating impossible spaces, and interacting with abstract concepts in a tangible way can lead to surprising discoveries. The brain, freed from the limitations of the waking world, begins to function in a more fluid and innovative way, providing experiences that can influence how the dreamer approaches creative challenges in real life.

Maintaining a detailed dream journal is crucial for capturing and making the most of these experiences. Many brilliant ideas may seem clear within the dream but quickly dissipate upon waking. Immediately jotting down any insight, scene, or creative concept allows these inspirations to be recorded and later developed in waking life.

Exploring creativity and problem-solving within lucid dreams transforms each dream experience into a unique opportunity for learning and innovation. Whether it's to improve a skill, seek artistic inspiration, or solve a practical dilemma, the dream world offers an infinite territory of possibilities. The dreamer who learns to consciously navigate this space can unlock profound aspects of their own mind, bringing to reality new ways of thinking, creating, and solving challenges.

Chapter 29
Spiritual Exploration in Dreams

The human consciousness possesses layers that transcend everyday experience, and lucid dreams reveal themselves as a powerful gateway to expanded states of perception. Upon awakening within the dream, the individual encounters a vast and limitless territory, where the boundaries between the real and the symbolic become fluid. In this space, existential questions can be explored in a profound way, revealing insights that escape the logical thinking of waking life. Since time immemorial, spiritual traditions have seen dreams as portals to other dimensions of being, a means of communication with subtler aspects of reality, and even a tool for reaching higher levels of consciousness. When the dreamer gains lucidity and directs their experience with intention, they can delve into this transformative potential, accessing hidden teachings and expanding their understanding of themselves and the universe.

Among the most striking experiences reported by those who use lucid dreams for spiritual exploration is the encounter with figures of wisdom. These characters, often described as masters, guides, or luminous beings, seem to possess a knowledge that transcends the dreamer's own. Dialogue with these entities can bring profound advice, enigmatic answers, or simply the feeling of contact with something greater. Furthermore, many practitioners experience moments of intense peace and connection, where the sense of individuality dissolves, giving way to a broadened perception of existence. This experience of unity, similar to the deepest meditative states, suggests that dreams can serve as a bridge between the personal mind and a larger consciousness, whether it is interpreted as spiritual, cosmic, or simply a deeper level of the psyche.

Another fascinating facet of spiritual exploration in lucid dreams is the sensation of passing through portals and accessing unknown realities. Some dreamers describe entering grandiose temples, ethereal cities, or landscapes of indescribable beauty, which seem to contain a silent wisdom. Others report encounters with deceased loved ones, experiences that can provide comfort and clarification about the continuity of existence. Whatever the interpretation of these experiences—as manifestations of the unconscious, mystical experiences, or journeys to other planes—they leave deep marks on the dreamer's perception. In this way, lucid dreams become not only a space for inner exploration, but also a tool for expanding the boundaries of known reality, leading the individual to new ways of understanding themselves and the mystery of existence.

One of the most common forms of spiritual seeking in lucid dreams is the encounter with guides or masters. Many people report that, upon becoming aware within a dream, they encounter figures who seem to possess superior wisdom. These guides may appear in the form of elders, beings of light, symbolic animals, or even familiar figures, such as teachers and mentors. For those who wish to experience this type of encounter, the key lies in intention. Before falling asleep, it's possible to program the mind to seek a meaningful encounter within the dream, formulating a clear request, such as: "I want to meet a guide who can teach me something important." Upon becoming lucid, simply reinforce this intention and allow the experience to unfold naturally.

Another frequently reported experience within spiritual lucid dreams is the sensation of unity and the dissolution of the ego. Some dreamers describe moments when the entire structure of the dream disappears, leaving only a vastness of light, a deep feeling of peace, or a pure consciousness without a defined form. This experience resembles deep meditative states and can bring a sense of connection with something greater, regardless of the dreamer's individual beliefs. In traditions such as Tibetan Buddhism, this experience is considered a glimpse of the true nature of the mind, a state beyond the illusions and projections of the material world.

The possibility of using lucid dreams to seek answers to existential questions is also a fascinating aspect of this journey. Within the dream, the dreamer can formulate questions directly to the dream universe, such as: "What is the purpose of my life?" or "What do I need to learn at this moment?". The answers can emerge in unexpected ways, whether through the speech of characters, symbols, or events that happen throughout the dream. The most interesting thing is that these answers often bring insights that the dreamer might not be able to access consciously in the waking state.

Some people also report experiences they interpret as encounters with deceased loved ones. Within the dream, these figures often appear full of peace and offer messages of comfort or farewell. Although there are various possible explanations for this phenomenon—from projections of the subconscious to the possibility of genuine contact, depending on each person's beliefs—the fact is that these interactions are usually emotionally impactful and leave a lasting sense of connection and understanding.

The sensation of passing through portals or visiting other realities is also a recurring theme among those who explore lucid dreams with a spiritual eye. Some people report entering grandiose temples, unknown cities, or landscapes that seem to exist beyond the world imagined by the dreamer himself. There are reports of encounters with unknown beings, access to libraries of infinite knowledge, or even experiences of flying through space, feeling part of the universe. For those who believe in realities beyond the physical, these journeys can be interpreted as explorations of other dimensional planes. For those who prefer a more psychological view, they are profound manifestations of imagination and the psyche. Whatever the interpretation, these experiences tend to leave a striking impression on the dreamer's mind.

The practice of setting spiritual intentions before sleep can increase the frequency of this type of dream. Praying, meditating, or simply mentalizing a sincere desire for learning before falling asleep creates a mental state conducive to these experiences occurring. Furthermore, during the dream, cultivating an attitude of respect and humility before the events can make the interactions deeper and more meaningful.

Lucid dreams offer a limitless territory for exploring the inner self and the great questions of existence. Whether in the search for answers, in the encounter with guides, or in the direct experience of pure consciousness, this practice allows the dreamer to expand their perception of reality and what it means to be awake, both inside and outside of dreams. What is found in this space varies according to the mind and beliefs of each individual, but one thing is certain: those who venture down this path rarely return the same.

Chapter 30
Tibetan Dream Yoga in Practice

The practice of Dream Yoga, present in Tibetan traditions for millennia, offers a profound path of self-discovery and spiritual development, going far beyond the simple experience of having awareness within dreams. Unlike the modern approach to lucid dreaming, which often focuses on dream control and creative exploration, this tradition emphasizes lucidity as a means to awaken to the true nature of mind and reality. In Tantric Buddhism and the Bön tradition, dreams are seen as manifestations of consciousness itself, and learning to navigate them with mindfulness can lead to liberation from the illusions that limit perception in the waking state. In this way, the practice not only enhances clarity within dreams but also strengthens presence and discernment in everyday life, promoting a continuous state of attention and wisdom.

The foundation of Dream Yoga lies in the understanding that waking reality and dreams share an essential characteristic: both are impermanent and shaped by the mind. Just as we accept unreal scenarios during sleep without questioning them, we often react mechanically to life's events, trapped in automatic patterns of thought and emotion. Dream training seeks to break this habitual unconsciousness, teaching the practitioner to recognize the fluidity of existence and the changing nature of experience. By developing lucidity in dreams, one exercises the ability to remain awake in waking life as well, perceiving events with greater clarity and reducing the suffering caused by attachment and aversion. This process leads to a state of expanded presence, in which reality is no longer experienced as an uncontrollable flow of events, but as a space of consciousness where it is possible to act with greater balance and discernment.

Beyond enhancing lucidity, the practice involves a progressive deepening in the exploration of the mind. Advanced techniques include completely dissolving the dream to experience pure awareness, deliberately modifying one's own form, or interacting with dream characters as spiritual teachers. These experiences are considered valuable preparations for the moment of death, when, according to Tibetan teachings, consciousness enters an intermediate state similar to a dream. One who has learned to maintain lucidity in dreams would be better able to navigate this transition with clarity and serenity. Thus, Dream Yoga is not just a dream practice, but a path to enlightenment, training the mind to recognize its true nature and free itself from the illusions that bind it to suffering.

The basis of this tradition is the idea that everyday reality is not so different from dreams. Just as in the dream state, we accept unreal scenarios without question, in the waking state we often react automatically to events, without realizing that we are immersed in a mental construct. By developing lucidity in dreams, the practitioner trains their mind to be equally awake in everyday life, recognizing the impermanence of experiences and the influence of one's own mind on reality.

The first steps of this practice involve cultivating dream recall and developing lucidity in a systematic way. Techniques such as keeping a dream journal and performing reality checks throughout the day are fundamental tools for strengthening dream awareness. In addition, Tibetan teachings emphasize the importance of cultivating a clear intention before sleep. During the period before sleep, the practitioner can meditate on the impermanence of the world or mentally repeat a mantra, reinforcing the determination to recognize the dream when it occurs.

Once lucid within the dream, the next stage of the practice involves maintaining stability and consciously observing dream phenomena without being carried away by distractions or intense emotions. Instead of trying to control the dream or shape it to one's own will, the practitioner is encouraged to remain aware of the experience without becoming attached to it, recognizing its illusory nature. This process strengthens the ability to maintain a state of presence and mindfulness, both in dreams and in waking life.

Another important aspect of Dream Yoga is deliberate experimentation with the dream environment to deepen understanding of the mind. The practitioner may try to pass through objects, change shape, or even completely dissolve the scenery around them, observing what happens when all images disappear. In some traditions, it is believed that this dissolution of the dream leads to a state of pure awareness, similar to that experienced during deep meditation.

In addition to exploring dreams themselves, Dream Yoga connects to a broader practice that involves maintaining a state of lucidity throughout the day. The concept of "daydreaming" is fundamental within this tradition, encouraging the practitioner to constantly question the nature of reality and cultivate a state of continuous presence. This training strengthens awareness not only in dreams but also in waking life, allowing the mind to become clearer and more balanced in the face of everyday challenges.

Within Tibetan Buddhism, it is believed that this practice also prepares the mind for death and the intermediate state known as bardo. Just as in a dream, the transition between life and death is seen as a moment of great mental malleability, where consciousness can be influenced by deep habits and patterns. One who has learned to maintain lucidity in dreams would, according to this view, be more prepared to navigate this transition with clarity and awareness.

The methods of Dream Yoga involve not only practical techniques but also mental training based on discipline and intention. In addition to keeping a dream journal and setting intentions before sleep, the practitioner can adopt visualization exercises, imagining themselves within a dream while awake, reinforcing the connection between waking and sleeping states. The repetition of specific mantras before falling asleep is also a central element of the tradition, helping to direct the mind towards a state of natural lucidity.

The application of this practice in everyday life goes beyond lucid dreaming. Continuous training to recognize the illusory nature of experiences leads to a greater lightness in the face of events, reducing the suffering caused by attachment and aversion. The perception of life as a dream does not mean denying its importance, but rather learning to interact with it in a more conscious and balanced way.

Those who dedicate themselves to this discipline often report an increase in mental clarity, intuition, and a sense of connection with something greater. Whether viewed as a spiritual practice or simply as a way to deepen understanding of the mind, the fact is that Dream Yoga offers a unique path to expand consciousness and transform the way we live both within dreams and beyond them.

Chapter 31
Out-of-Body Experiences

Out-of-body experiences (OBEs) represent one of the most intriguing phenomena in the exploration of human consciousness, challenging the boundaries between subjective perception and objective reality. Accounts throughout history, stemming from diverse spiritual traditions and modern investigations, indicate that consciousness can temporarily dissociate from the physical body, allowing the individual a vivid sensation of displacement to different environments, dimensions, or states of existence. This unique experience is often described with impressive realism, providing a sharp sensory perception and, often, a profound emotional and philosophical impact. While some people experience this separation spontaneously, others seek specific methods to induce it, whether through meditative techniques, deep relaxation, or practices related to lucid dreaming. The fascination with this phenomenon lies both in the experience itself and in its implications, which challenge established conceptions about the mind, consciousness, and the very nature of reality.

The distinction between astral projection and advanced oneiric states, such as lucid dreaming, is a widely debated issue among scholars of the subject and experienced practitioners. While lucid dreams occur within an oneiric context recognizably shaped by the subconscious, out-of-body experiences are frequently described as events of expanded perception, in which the individual has the clear impression of interacting with an environment independent of their own mind. Many report observing their sleeping body from an external point of view, moving through familiar or unknown spaces, and, in some cases, encountering presences or entities that appear to have their own existence. These descriptions lead some researchers to consider the possibility that the phenomenon is more than a brain construct, suggesting that it may involve aspects of human consciousness not yet understood. However, traditional science tends to explain these experiences as manifestations of altered states of perception, influenced by neurological processes such as sleep paralysis, hypnagogic hallucinations, and the dynamics of the cerebral cortex during the transition between wakefulness and sleep.

Regardless of the explanations, the subjective experience of out-of-body projections has a profound impact on those who experience them. Many report an intense sense of freedom, an expansion of perception, and, in some cases, transformations in their worldview and personal beliefs. For some, astral projection represents a genuine spiritual journey, a means of accessing hidden knowledge or exploring realities beyond the physical plane. For others, it is a field of psychological exploration, where the study of consciousness reveals new layers of the human mind.

Whatever the interpretation, out-of-body experiences continue to intrigue, inspire, and challenge the conventional understanding of reality, encouraging those interested in the subject to deepen their research and practice, exploring the mysteries of consciousness with an open mind and critical discernment.

The main difference between lucid dreams and out-of-body experiences lies in the perception of reality during the event. In a lucid dream, the dreamer realizes they are dreaming, but generally recognizes that the surrounding environment is a creation of the subconscious. In astral projection, the sensation is often of total separation from the physical body, accompanied by intense sensory clarity and the impression of being in an environment that exists independently of the projector's mind. This state often begins with peculiar sensations, such as vibrations throughout the body, a buzzing in the ears, or the impression of being pulled out of oneself.

Many reports of astral projection begin in the intermediate phase between sleep and wakefulness, especially when the person awakens in the middle of the night but keeps the body relaxed and still. Sensations of floating, temporary paralysis, or even the impression of spinning on one's own axis are common before the supposed separation of consciousness. Some describe a moment of transition where they feel themselves getting out of bed and observing their own sleeping body, which reinforces the belief that they are indeed outside the physical body.

One of the greatest difficulties for those seeking this type of experience is fear. The sensation of detachment can be intense and unexpected, leading many to wake up abruptly before completing the separation. The fear of not being able to return to the body or of encountering unknown presences can block the process. However, those who delve deeper into this practice often report that the experience is safe and controllable, and that the intention to return to the body is enough for it to occur instantly.

Navigation during astral projection is reported to be different from that in lucid dreams. Many claim that, instead of walking or consciously manipulating the scenery, they move through intention, simply thinking of a destination to be transported to it. Some describe visits to known places, while others claim to access unknown environments, such as mysterious cities, temples, or interdimensional landscapes. There are also reports of encounters with entities or beings that seem to have their own consciousness, which raises questions about the nature of the plane they are in.

Interpretations of astral projection vary widely. Some spiritual traditions claim that consciousness actually separates from the physical body and travels to other planes of existence. From a scientific point of view, there are alternative explanations, such as the hypothesis that these experiences are altered states of consciousness generated by the brain, similar to hypnagogic hallucinations or an advanced form of lucid dreaming. Studies suggest that certain areas of the brain related to the perception of space and the body can create the illusion of being outside oneself, especially in states of deep relaxation or during sleep paralysis.

Regardless of the explanation, what matters to the practitioner is the experience itself. Many report that projections bring a profound sense of freedom, introspection, and expansion of consciousness. For those who wish to experience this phenomenon, some techniques can be applied. Staying calm when feeling the initial vibrations, avoiding moving the physical body when perceiving the transition, and focusing on the intention to project are recommended practices. In addition, visualizing a desired location or repeating a mental command, such as "Now I will project myself," can help induce the experience.

Those who explore lucid dreams often wonder if out-of-body experiences are just a deeper level of oneiric lucidity or if they actually represent something more. Although there is no definitive consensus, the reality is that both phenomena can be trained and improved, allowing the practitioner to expand their perception and discover, on their own, the limits and possibilities of consciousness. The important thing is to keep an open mind, record the experiences, and explore this unknown territory with curiosity and discernment, allowing each journey to offer new learnings and insights into the very nature of reality.

Chapter 32
Integrating Dream and Reality

Awakened consciousness reaches its full potential when it transcends the boundaries of sleep and expands into wakefulness, transforming everyday perception into a continuous state of lucidity. The same questioning gaze that enables the experience of lucid dreaming can be directed toward waking reality, fostering a deeper understanding of one's own existence. Life, often lived on autopilot, becomes a field of active exploration, where each moment carries richer meaning and each experience can be shaped by conscious attention. Integrating the lucidity of dreams into daily life means living with greater presence, recognizing automatic patterns of thought, and developing a more intentional relationship with one's own mind. This process enables not only an expansion of perception but also a genuine transformation in how one interacts with the world.

The relationship between dream and reality is more fluid than it appears, as both are constructs of consciousness and depend on how they are interpreted. In the dream state, the mind creates scenarios and events spontaneously, responding to the dreamer's emotions and thoughts. Similarly, in the waking state, perceptions are filtered by internal beliefs, expectations, and conditioning, shaping each individual's experience. By perceiving this influence of the mind on reality, it becomes possible to question automatic patterns and adopt a more active stance towards life. Small changes in perception can modify how challenges are faced, how interpersonal relationships are experienced, and how the very meaning of existence is revealed. When lucidity transcends the limits of the dream and permeates everyday life, the experience of reality becomes more plastic, dynamic, and accessible to conscious influence.

Integrating dream lucidity and waking consciousness doesn't just mean recognizing similarities between dream and wakefulness, but rather using the lessons learned in lucid dreams to transform the way one lives. The sense of control and creativity experienced in dreams can be applied to the search for innovative solutions, overcoming emotional blocks, and building a more authentic and meaningful life. The practice of questioning reality, maintaining mindfulness, and observing one's own mind without identifying with automatic thoughts enables a continuous state of presence. Life, previously perceived as rigid and predictable, reveals itself to be malleable and full of possibilities, allowing each individual to take on a more conscious role in the construction of their own journey.

Most people live on autopilot, reacting to events without deeply questioning the nature of their experiences. Just as in dreams we accept absurd events without questioning them, in waking life we often go through situations without truly paying attention, absorbed in automatic thoughts and distractions. The practice of lucidity proposes a different approach, based on mindfulness and the recognition of the impermanence of experiences.

One of the first steps to integrate the teachings of lucid dreams into wakefulness is to cultivate the same curiosity and critical sense that awaken consciousness within dreams. Regularly questioning "Am I dreaming?" throughout the day not only increases the chance of achieving lucidity in dreams but also teaches the mind to observe reality more clearly. This practice develops a deeper state of presence, where each moment is lived more consciously and deliberately.

Observing mental and emotional patterns is also an essential tool for living more lucidly. In dreams, emotions directly influence the scenery and events. Similarly, in wakefulness, thoughts and emotional states shape the perception of reality. A person who constantly finds themselves caught up in negative or anxious thoughts will experience a world filtered through those emotions. Developing the ability to recognize and question these patterns allows for greater freedom and control over how one responds to life's challenges.

The creativity and mental flexibility cultivated in lucid dreams can also be brought into wakefulness. In the dream world, the dreamer discovers that they can alter scenarios, overcome obstacles, and create impossible experiences. Although the laws of the physical world are more rigid, the mind remains the primary tool for interpreting reality. When one learns to see life as a space for experimentation, it becomes easier to find innovative solutions to problems, deal with changes more adaptably, and see opportunities where there were once limitations.

The practice of gratitude and appreciation for the present moment is also strengthened by lucidity training. Many people who begin to have lucid dreams report a newfound admiration for the waking world, perceiving details previously ignored, sensing more vivid colors, and connecting with the small wonders of everyday life. This state of presence and enchantment can be consciously cultivated, making each experience more meaningful.

Another important aspect of lucid living is self-knowledge. Dreams reveal much about the psyche, bringing to the surface desires, fears, and internal patterns. Similarly, wakefulness can be used as a mirror to better understand who we are. Observing reactions, analyzing recurring thoughts, and seeking the cause of emotions can lead to a deeper level of understanding and personal transformation.

The idea that reality is as malleable as dreams doesn't mean that the physical world can be manipulated in the same way as a dreamscape, but rather that the perception of life can be adjusted as consciousness expands. When a person realizes that their mind directly influences their experience of the world, they become more responsible for their own reality, learning to direct their attention and energy to what they want to create.

Living lucidly doesn't just mean seeking extraordinary experiences in dreams, but rather awakening to the depth and richness of one's own existence. Every moment can be lived with more presence, every challenge can be faced with more awareness, and every choice can be made in a way that is more aligned with what truly matters. The practice of lucid dreaming is an invitation to see life in a more awakened way, recognizing that, just as in dreams, we are the creators of our own journey.

Chapter 33
Dream Mastery and Next Steps

The exploration of lucid dreaming reaches its true meaning when it transforms into a continuous journey of self-discovery, transcending mere curiosity and becoming a powerful tool for personal growth. The awareness gained in dream states not only reveals the hidden mechanisms of the mind but also teaches valuable lessons about perception, control, and the nature of reality. With each lucid experience, the practitioner deepens their relationship with the subconscious, unlocks creative potential, and expands their understanding of the self. Dream mastery is not a goal to be achieved, but a constantly evolving process, where each night represents a new opportunity for learning and experimentation. Instead of viewing dream mastery as an end, it should be seen as an invitation to explore the mysteries of consciousness with curiosity, discipline, and openness to the unexpected.

Continuous practice of lucid dreaming requires a balance between technique and spontaneity, allowing the experience to unfold naturally without rigid impositions. Maintaining a dream journal remains an essential strategy, as it helps strengthen dream recall and identify patterns that can be used to induce lucidity.

Furthermore, cultivating mindfulness in waking life strengthens the habit of questioning reality, expanding the ability to recognize the moments when one is dreaming. For those seeking to deepen their knowledge, exchanging experiences with other lucid dreamers can offer new perspectives and motivation to continue advancing. Forums, study groups, and shared accounts help diversify approaches and overcome common challenges on the journey of lucidity.

The paths to explore the potential of lucid dreams are varied and adaptable to individual interests. Some may use them as a source of artistic inspiration, transforming dream images and narratives into music, painting, or literature. Others may focus on therapeutic application, exploring traumas and emotional challenges in a safe and malleable environment. There are also those who see lucid dreams as a spiritual tool, a means of accessing expanded states of consciousness and deepening their connection with more subtle aspects of existence. Regardless of the purpose, the experience of lucidity in dreams transcends the night, directly influencing how one lives the day. The awareness gained in the dream world is reflected in waking reality, making it more vibrant, meaningful, and amenable to transformation. The dreamer who understands this connection realizes that true mastery is not just about controlling dreams, but about using this knowledge to awaken, more deeply, to one's own life.

Dream mastery is not a final destination, but an ongoing process of discovery. Each night brings new opportunities to explore the mind and deepen the connection with the subconscious. Some people will easily achieve lucidity frequently, while others will need more time to hone their skills. The key is to keep the practice alive, even in periods when lucid dreams seem less frequent. Consistency is the key to making lucidity a natural and recurring phenomenon.

Maintaining a dream journal will continue to be one of the most valuable habits on this journey. The simple act of recording nightly experiences strengthens dream recall and allows one to recognize recurring patterns, facilitating the induction of lucidity. In addition, reviewing previous entries can bring valuable insights into emotional and psychological changes over time, transforming the dream journal into a true map of the subconscious mind.

The development of mindfulness in waking life also continues to be an essential factor in the evolution of the practice. The more aware you are during the day, the easier it will be to carry this clarity into the dream state. The practice of presence, of observing thoughts, and of questioning reality not only increases the frequency of lucid dreams but also improves the quality of life, reducing the feeling of living on autopilot and bringing more meaning to everyday experiences.

For those who wish to deepen their studies even further, exploring communities of lucid dreamers can be an enriching experience. Forums, discussion groups, and meetings on the subject bring together people who share the same interest and who can offer tips, reports, and new perspectives on the practice. Sharing experiences and learning from other practitioners helps to maintain motivation and to discover approaches that may not have been considered before.

The exploration of dreams can follow different paths, depending on the interests of each individual. Some may wish to focus on creativity, using lucid dreams as a source of inspiration for artistic, musical, or literary projects. Others may deepen the therapeutic aspect, working through repressed emotions and using the dream environment to overcome inner fears and challenges. There are also those who are attracted to the spiritual dimension of the experience, using lucid dreams as a means of advanced meditation, the search for meaning, or even the exploration of altered states of consciousness.

Regardless of the goal, the most efficient approach is always the one that balances discipline and lightness. Forcing lucidity or turning dreams into an obligation can create anxiety and harm the experience. The best path is to maintain an attitude of curiosity and experimentation, allowing dreams to unfold naturally while applying the techniques learned. Some nights will be more intense and full of lucidity, others will bring little or no memory, but each of them is part of the improvement process.

The connection between dreams and waking life becomes increasingly evident as the practice advances. Just as in the dream world, where awareness allows one to modify scenarios and interact with events in an active way, waking reality can also be transformed as one develops greater control over thoughts, emotions, and actions. The perception of life as a dynamic flow of possibilities is strengthened, allowing each person to become not only a master of their own dreams, but also a conscious creator of their own reality.

The journey towards dream mastery is just beginning. Every night is a new opportunity to explore, learn and grow. Every awakening, a chance to apply the lessons learned in dreams to live with more presence and authenticity. The path continues, and the dreamer who has understood its potential will never see their own dreams—and their own life—in the same way.

Epilogue

And so, what remains when the lights of the dream fade and the eyes awaken to wakefulness? What remains when the dream universe dissolves into the ethereal and we return to the familiar stage of waking reality?

You have embarked on a deep journey through the vast territory of consciousness. You have traveled through the mysteries of lucid dreams, explored the techniques of the ancients and of modern science, learned to distinguish illusion from reality, and, perhaps, have felt firsthand the incomparable ecstasy of awakening within a dream. But now, as you reach the end of these pages, the question that echoes is not about what has been learned, but about what will be done with this knowledge.

Dreams have always been there, whispering hidden truths while you slept. But now, you can see them with new eyes. Now, you know that they are not just ephemeral images that dissolve at dawn. They are mirrors, portals, powerful tools that shape not only the nights, but also the days. For what happens in the dream realm does not remain isolated—it reverberates in the core of the mind, reconfigures beliefs, undoes fears, and opens doors to a deeper understanding of who we are.

The one who masters their dreams not only controls a nightly fantasy—they shape their own reality. For the mind that awakens within the dream is the same that awakens to life. If in dreams we can defy the laws of physics, transcend limitations, and manifest will, then what prevents us from applying this same principle to the waking world?

The limit has always been in belief.

And belief can be transformed.

The understanding of the dream universe teaches us that reality is more flexible than we imagine. That what we judge to be immutable can, in fact, be shaped. If within a lucid dream we can learn to transform fear into courage, doubt into conviction, and flight into mastery, then why can't we do the same with our lives?

The practice of lucid dreaming is not just a tool for living impossible adventures, but a training for consciousness. It is an expansion of being, an invitation to question self-imposed limitations, an opportunity to integrate wakefulness and sleep into a continuous state of mindfulness. When we understand that we are creators within the dream, we begin to suspect that we are also creators outside of it.

And that is the great revelation.

The barrier between the real and the illusory is thinner than we think. Just as we learn to question the nature of dreams, we can learn to question the stories we tell ourselves about our own existence. What we accept as absolute truth may be as mutable as a dreamscape. What we were told was impossible may prove to be just a misguided belief.

You now possess the keys. You know how to awaken in the dream and take control. But there is an even greater awakening awaiting you: the one that happens within your own life.

Reality is not fixed.
The mind is infinite.
And the dream...
The dream never ends.

It unfolds with every night, every thought, every choice. It continues, whether you are sleeping or walking through the waking world. For those who learn to dream consciously also learn to live consciously.

And this is just the beginning.

www.ingramcontent.com/pod-product-compliance
Lightning Source LLC
LaVergne TN
LVHW040056080526
838202LV00045B/3668